How I Defeated Death from Lyme and West-Nile

The Lord's Guidance In My Ability to Defeating
Death from Lyme and West Nile

KATHY GAA

PAGE PUBLISHING, INC.
Conneaut Lake, PA

First originally published by Page Publishing 2020

ISBN 978-1-64701-773-6 (pbk)
ISBN 978-1-64701-775-0 (digital)

Printed in the United States of America

CONTENTS

INTRODUCTION

The year is 2018.

I am writing this book to share with you my experiences and the battles I have had and how I am now finally winning the battle with Lyme and West Nile. I was and finally I am able to see more clearly just how God has used these diseases and the paths he directed me on to meet the gifted instructors, doctors, as well as those naturally gifted healers who also came into my life that helped in so many ways, which in turn helped me to inspire, and offer help to others on their path to healing.

There are various challenges and troubles each and every one of us has to encounter in life. You will sometimes discover that people show concern toward assisting you. As lovely as this may possibly sound, you are the only one that can take that first step towards helping yourself.

That is, if you actually care enough to begin the journey to help yourself.

This is my story, and I pray it will be an inspiration to live a healthier life. Thank you for this time to share in your life!

CHAPTER ONE

My Story

Just after starting my massage classes, I was offered a job in an alternative care clinic that taught me so much through all the positives and negatives (as there are in any situation), I am so very fortunate to have learned so much.

While working there for six and a half years, I had the privileged of doing treatments using the modalities I had learned through my massage courses. People would come from all over the country, who were suffering with all forms of issues. While working in the clinic, I had the opportunity of using and becoming more familiar with essential oils to the point of developing my own face cream that people who used it would claim tell me *"it's magic."* So I decided to call it ***"Facial Magic,"*** which you can learn more about and order by going to my website.

I was also learning more about live blood and dark-field microscopy work. From there, I started comparing the blood work with how the client's feet looked and the skin felt, as well as the intensity of tenderness while giving reflexology treatments. So from there, depending on where the tenderness was on the feet, would clue me in to what the blood work was showing. As my experience grew from doing reflexology for the clients, I began to clue in more and more to the different levels of tenderness in certain areas, on the feet that would suggest, just how much that person was suffering, from Lyme or West Nile.

So while I was still working in the clinic, the clients started asking me to do more treatments for them. For the type of treatments (modalities) I was doing, I learned they gave the clients such great relief from their pain and suffering, which enabled me to become more sure about how successful these treatments worked for others as they did for me.

Later, I moved to Wyoming, where I have been using the modalities I put together to help my own clientele who were suffering and who also had been unsuccessful in finding any relief from their pain and illness.

As I mentioned before, I started to gain a realization that these methods helped those who suffered from these ailments. I want to explain how that realization came into fruition and how it progressed into the program I use now.

There was a massage therapist, whom I will call El, who started working in the clinic with me and had training in similar modalities that I had been trained in. From there, we shared our knowledge and began putting modalities and ideas together. The two modalities we had both learned from our classes were acupressure and polarity balancing. This is what got our imaginations going.

The first time El did an acupressure treatment for auto-immune disease for me, was miraculous! I discovered through the blood work research (microscopy) that I had Lyme disease. And this is how I discovered I had been suffering from Lyme for thirty years! I had symptoms of fibromyalgia so painful that I had *to take way too much,* of a popular over the counter pain medicine in order to function at all! Even though I was taking all those pain meds, they still did not even come close to subsiding the pain I was experiencing twenty-four hours a day, seven days a week. I did not consider even taking prescription meds and take a chance of becoming addicted and/or becoming afflicted with the possible side effects they are known to cause for I had enough to deal with!

I will take a step back to shed some light on how much the acupressure treatment helped me. Halfway through El performing treatment, I had an epiphany where I thought, *If I had this treatment done every day for six weeks, I would be healed!* This sudden thought was put into action and *all my pain* was dissipating! When she finished the treatment, *I was totally out of pain*! I haven't been free of pain since the toxemia with my first son (who will be forty-one years old this year).

Then within an hour after the treatment, I started feeling my energy increase and continued to do so as the day went on. So after arriving back to my apartment after work, guess what I did? I used that energy that I hadn't felt since my last lifetime (so to speak, LOL) to catch up on things I hadn't been able to do for so long, I can't even remember when! Well, I found out soon that that was a mistake for the very next day, I was tired, although I was still out of pain. I knew then I should have rested and used that extra energy for healing, rather than catching up on things due to using the energy I gained from the treatment. It was about three to four more treatment before I could gain that same energy back again! And yes, you could say I was pretty discouraged to say the least! ***But that's how I learned just how important it is to rest as much as possible to allow the extra energy to go to healing instead of spending it on foolishness (I will say).*** As for the pain, it didn't return for three days! AMAZING! I was on top of the world then for I had found a treatment that eliminated, not only my pain but, also at the same time built my energy levels up! I will say again, **"THAT'S AMAZING!"**

El wasn't the only one who helped me with those many treatments. My dear friends Kassia, Kimberly (mentioned in Ch.6), and Noramae Craig (who has been like a mother and mentor in my life) my dear friend Kassia would also perform the treatments for me. After having a few of these acupressure treatments, I was amazed how my body was responding. To my surprise, I found that when I would give others the same acupressure treatment, they too experienced the same responses as I did. *I started realizing the trick is to retrain the body's energy to hold on its own and, in order to achieve those results, is to have this treatment done at least every two days and up to even once or twice a day for a week maybe two. Then as time goes, then the treatments can become further apart depending on how chronic the Lyme or West Nile is for each individual person.*

CHAPTER TWO

West Nile versus Basil Essential Oil

I also found the use of certain essential oils extremely helpful as well. I found after contracting West Nile, that I was craving basil essential oil, and due to the migraines, neck, and spine aches that seem to accompany West Nile, I found when I applied the basil oil, to the back of the neck, the migraine, and neck ache would dissipate within seconds!

So I started applying it to the people who were suffering from the symptoms of West Nile they all had the same reactions as I did when I would apply the basil oil to their neck. The people I would do essential oil treatments for, who were suffering with West Nile, I found they would come back the next day to purchase all the oils I used on them, saying that was the only thing that took the pain away!

CHAPTER THREE

My Secret Weapon: Essential Oil, "Weapon" Recipe for Lyme and West Nile

Here is the inspired list of essential oils I use to relieve pain caused from the West Nile virus.

Black pepper 3 drops, 3 drops oregano (a hot oil…used for virus and bacteria infections), 3 drops clove (a hot oil…used for pain relief), 6 drops peppermint (to help heal the nerves). The peppermint will also give a cooling sensation after it finishes working, so apply the peppermint last. And black pepper essential oil is one of my favorite oils to use that penetrates deep into the muscles creating a warm soothing, and relaxing sensation.

Caution: *Never add hot or warming oils to a bath! They can give a person acid burns! Always use a carrier oil with along with these hotter oils.*

Eucalyptus 8 drops (for pain and inflammation), rosemary 8 drops (for circulation, autoimmune diseases, and an antibiotic), lavender 8 drops (to relax the muscle spasms that the West Nile may cause), and then of course, basil 8 drops. (:

After applying the oils, I heat up a bath towel with hot water, which I would wring the water out *JUST enough so it was not drip-*

ping any water. Then I ***slowly apply the towel*** by starting on the low back and then lower it slowly down onto the rest of the back to cover the shoulders and neck. If the person was tall, I would apply a smaller towel to the neck. Next, I apply a dry bath towel over the wet ones, for thirty minutes. *By leaving the towels on for thirty minutes, this will also help balance the energies of the body for healing.*

In the palm of my hand I mix all of the essential oils I intend to use, with a bit of carrier oil, ***(except the peppermint oil, which I apply last)***, by stirring in a clock wise motion, with one of my fingers, I then apply to the back, neck and shoulders. After applying the mixture of oils, I apply the peppermint oil. The reason for this is, you will feel the different oils as they work in the order you apply them. Therefore as the peppermint oil begins to work you will start to feel a cooling effect in spots that will progress till your whole back has a cooling sensation. That's when I slowly remove the damp towels with a follow up of a dry towel which I leave on till the coolness subsides.

In the order that you apply the oils is the order in which each one takes their turn to work. Again, this is why you will want to apply the peppermint oil last.

The amounts I use varies, depending on the individual and on how sensitive their skin is. If they have sensitive skin, which most people with very fair complexions tend to have, then go very easy on the amount of oils you use by using less drops. The oils will heat up due to pulling toxins. If they get too warm, apply a carrier oil, by lifting the towels only slightly to apply the oil, this can be olive oil, coconut oil, avocado oil, or any oil as long as you do not have an allergy to it. As soon as the oil is applied, the area will cool off.

If you do not have time to do the treatment or just need something on your aches and pains, you can mix up a smaller batch and apply. ***For just aches and pains, I don't add the oregano oil. I find it gets to hot and it's not the kind of hot you want for aches and pains.***

I also do an oil pulling for my gums. I first brush my teeth, then mix 2 to 3 drops of rosemary essential oil in water. Before brushing my teeth I add a couple of drops of rosemary to my toothpaste. I find that rosemary essential oil seems to kill the spirochetes that can harbor in the gums and cause soreness in them as well as, also may cause the teeth to decay quite rapidly, which also happened to me within just a few short months of contacting West Nile. I have also seen this very same thing happen to other people's teeth as well.

I then soak and swish the mixture in my mouth for twenty minutes. Then brush my teeth.

JUST BE SURE TO _**NOT**_ USE LOTION AND OR WATER TO DILUTE DOWN THE ESSENTIAL OILS. THIS IS VERY IMPORTANT! It will cause the oils to get even hotter! I have actually seen this happen, one person even had, what looked like acid burns on his skin!

**WARNING: So keep a carrier oil at your fingertips when using essential oils AT ALL TIMES! USE all ESSENTIAL OILS WITH CAUTION!**

They are very strong and the hotter oils like oregano, black pepper, clove, lemon, lime, cinnamon, etcetera. _If you over use them, they can cause burns!_

**JUST BE SURE TO NOT USE LOTION TO THIN DOWN THE ESSENTIAL OILS.**

I highly recommend taking an essential oils class to become more familiar with the oils.

CHAPTER FOUR

Supplement Plan

At that time, I felt if I continued on the program of supplements that I was on at that time, I would recover. So, sticking on my path to recovery, I felt I should continue staying on the supplement program. Then a couple of years later while getting ready for work, I found my liver was drastically swollen! It was not just a little swollen, it was swollen clear out from under my ribs! My left side was normal. I'm thinking, *Okay, this is the end of me.* Then I heard a very loud prompting saying, "Stop taking the supplements! You will be okay."

So from there, I started putting two and two together realizing why I had started gaining weight and could not lose it. I had been able to keep my weight down for all those years after I lost weight from my last son (I have two sons) which I never weighed over 108 pounds and was always able to wear a size 5 western jeans. (At this time, I am not discussing my weight,) lols

I was also very agile as well, reminiscing back of how I was able to run up a flight of stairs if in a hurry. When putting it all together of my decline of not being able to keep the weight off, the loss of my agility, the right side of thyroid swelling up, losing all eyebrows, the worst part was I could not do a fast any more, for I would feel as though my blood sugar was going South! So, I would go for a checkup to see what it was doing but it was always in the normal range! It was even in the lower half of normal, so I just did not know where to go from there. I had started this type of decline around six months after I started taking a certain line of supplements. The odd thing was, my blood was showing improvement and the AcuGraph test (this measures your energy levels) started showing all green and good energy, but I wasn't feeling better! This was very disturbing to me.

Because everyone else who I worked on and that was having treatments in the clinic was healing up. So this just shows me that my doctor in Vegas I went to see long ago, was very familiar and who very much understood extra sensitive people such as myself, for he did warn me, of even being very careful of not only foods I ate, but supplements as well, he also warned me about the different injections that are available in alternative care clinics. That they could do me in. Do to being extra sensitive not just to foods, etc. But also to people and my surroundings. Thinking back, I needed to hang around him to learn more about myself because back when I was growing up, the word "sensitivity" just *did not* exist! LOLS! Being a farm girl, you had to be tough! If you were sick, you either died if the home remedy didn't work or got better! Yeah, you had a choice, back then. What more does a person need? lols! For something was amiss in those days, you think?

Since then after my move to Wyoming, I have tried a few other product lines like professional lines, and a very well-known pyramid line. One of my very dear (angel) friends, Kimberly, said after taking a look at the ingredients of the meal replacement product, "That it has peas and potato for its protein base which can cause you to gain weight!"

My reply was, "Well, I had started feeling better on it. The company had changed the formula some time since I had started taking it. I had not paid any attention to the ingredient list since it was helping me in the beginning." I had even started losing weight and my eyebrows were starting to grow back in, although I was still very tired and still experiencing much pain. Now I know why I had stopped improving.

This was just one of the paths the Lord has taken me down to show me just how taking something that is wrong for your body (whether it is a supplement brand or a food, drink, etcetera) can really throw your system off-balance.

More Discovery about What Essentials Oils to Use for West Nile

The summer I moved to Wyoming was when I contracted West Nile. Many people who had also contracted West Nile were also coming to the clinic for treatment. This is when I discovered what essential oils to use (as always) through the Spirit's promptings that would take the pain away so as to help encourage the healing process.

What I am about to share with you now is how I discovered what essential oils to use for the pain and illness that West Nile causes.

One morning after contracting West Nile while getting ready for work, my right elbow started hurting, it started to worsen by the second! When the pain escalated to a point that I could not even think of going to work, let alone drive! As always, the Spirit prompted me once again. I heard, ***"Slap on your rosemary essential oil and rub it into your elbows really well."*** So I did just that. To my surprise, the pain was stopped almost immediately! As soon as the pain was completely gone, which was in a matter of a few seconds, I was then told, ***"You see, the rosemary kills the West Nile and Lyme!"***

Miraculously, I was able to go to work!

CHAPTER FIVE

The Sci-Fi Experience

Not too long after that I moved back to Cody, Wyoming, and then to Powell, where I proceeded to build a very good practice, in which everyone that came to see me is just awesome and very special to me, and I am so grateful to have them all in my life. And I know that is very uncommon for such a thing to happen, so I feel very blessed.

The West Nile was affecting my lymphatic system to a great degree. Due to not being able to rest and have someone to do lymphatic draining for me for some time, and that's not to mention about the pressure of starting a business, and who only knew where it was going to go. So I began taking five capsules of rosemary every morning. I was also using my reflexology machine that has infra-red heat, and also my chi machine that helps to move lymphatics. Even with that the West Nile still progressed to the point that my right arm became twice as large as my left one, and my lymph nodes were swelling up as well *(some where the size of pullet eggs)* and becoming quite hard due to not draining sufficiently.

Another friend, who at that time, which happened to be chronically afflicted with Lyme was a great deal of help to me. She had found supplements on the internet that benefited her significantly. The supplements were Bio-Fibrin and Monolaurin. So I decided to try them as well. I must admit I wish I had actually discovered the Body Code and Systemic Formulas' protocol for Lyme disease instead. For with the Body Code program, I could've asked to see if there was a supplement program that was much better suited for my health issues and concerns. That's the whole aspect of trying to figure out and to identify what's going on yourself, sometimes a person simply doesn't know how to go about finding out everything that's available for their own specific health needs. Then there's word of mouth information, the thing about this is, what may be right for one person's health issues and sensitivities may not necessarily work for the next person. Another question you might want to ask…are there any substances in the formulas that you have an allergen or sensitive to. As was my experience where specific formulations and IV's happened to be quite caustic to my body. Be Aware! The vitamin C in some supplement and IV products are corn based! No wonder I say "that I gained weight since I have an allergen to corn!" And here's a reminder, and food for thought…corn is what they feed the animals to fatten them up. This is why I can't stress enough to those who do choose alternative care methods just how important it is to have someone who has training in muscle testing to make sure your body is okay with everything you choose to ingest as well as the treatments you plan to do for your body and this includes testing for the types of bodywork, machines, magnets, and yes, even for different types of exercises that you are considering on doing. In which I will expand on next. My reason for testing what type of exercises will most benefit your immediate health situation, when I found that whatever was plaguing me was in my own hands to deal with. I decided to do yoga, which I had been reading was great for everyone. So I decided to give it a try and even though I started off very slowly, it sat me back immensely in that I felt so ill I couldn't move for a couple of days. Now then I must tell you about how I did go outside in the fresh mountain air every day to walk, I also did a lot of horseback riding, and I for sure got a lot of exercising in, during hunting season by hiking in the mountains and horseback riding in the hills and especially during the two years when I was carrying five-gallon buckets full of water uphill sixty yards which happened to be up a fairly steep incline to the cabin most every day, before we were able to drill a well. And what's amazing…is that all of those activities never sat me back health wise as did the Yoga exercises. During that period of time in my life…if I could do more exercising designed for balancing one's chakras and energy fields my health would start to turn around rather than the slow decline in which I continued to experience. So with that being said, I happened to find books on Tibetan, Tai chi, and Qigong exercises, which surprisingly enough I was able to do those exercises without any setbacks. Once more, the reason I've felt strongly impressed to write this book is in the hope of boosting one's imagination to look into all the possibilities that are readily available to you.

After I started taking the Bio-Fibrin and Monolaurin along with taking the rosemary capsules as well, I did start noting a big change, but still not totally healing up completely, due to the scaring and damage these creatures leave behind. With this program we would compare notes on how we were progressing. What I'm about to share with you next is where my story starts sounding like a sci-fi fiction novel. Here goes…there were times we would feel as though something was moving or crawling under our scalps! Then in a matter of seconds we would start to feel a bit dizzy, and woozy to boot! We really had it going on! Ya think? Then the next day we would experience an itchy spot on our head, when we reached up to calm it down, that's when we would notice a scab had formed on our scalp in that particular area during the night. It was like these things were trying to work themselves out from underneath our scalps! It did how ever make our head quite sore at times. When these episodes started, it was quite tender, once again I had a prompting to just pour some rosemary on the area when I felt things moving. So I gave it a try, and to my amazement, it stopped moving and the tenderness went away!

Well, I have to share this one particular time when I felt something large move under my scalp at the crown of my head, plus it scared the heck out of me, to say the least! If that rosemary didn't kill it, I was OUT the door to the hospital, immediately! I'm thinking, *There goes the rest of my brain!* So I hurried and poured like a half a bottle of rosemary on my head—and it DID the job! The crawling instantly stopped! Thank the Lord! For, as you can imagine, what I was thinking, *What if the rosemary didn't work?* Like what would they do at the hospital to me? And would a specialist be around to help me out? We did find that we had to leave the scabs alone and continue to use the rosemary essential oil (due to the itching they created), for it, would heal better and faster. As this was all taking place, a few days later I had felt inclined to stop to see how another "angel friend": (of which I am blessed with many) was doing who just happened to live in a nostalgic cute trailer in Ralston just approximately twenty miles from Cody and only approximately four miles from Powell. The trailer house was right across the only gas/quick stop in town right on the main road from Cody to Powell. Imagine that!

I will stop here for a bit and back up to when I was working at the clinic when I contacted West Nile, I started noticing when I would do reflexology for people who were victimized by West Nile, *I began noticing my liver felt as though it was churning, which it would continue to do so 'til I stopped the reflexology treatment!* This happened every time I would do reflexology for someone who had West Nile!

After moving to Wyoming, I continued with my protocol, for several months which consisted of the rosemary capsules and applying the rosemary oil then with the addition of the Bio-Fibrin, and Monolaurin. That's when I noticed my liver had finally stopped churning when I would do reflexology treatments for anyone who had contacted West Nile. It was as though the spirochetes were communicating from one host to another! I know it all sounds pretty crazy! And believe me, I was beginning to think I was heading there! It was approximately year and a half of taking the rosemary capsules, monolaurin and the bio-fibrin before the spirochetes were gone and the episodes with my liver had stopped. I just wished I had found Systemic Formulas much sooner.

Although I still had a lot of healing to do from all the spiraling effects the spirochetes are known to do throughout the body. To this day I am not so sure if I will ever see a hundred percent healing, although the one thing is for sure is that I'm very grateful for having way more energy, and for no longer suffering from the constant horrific brain fog, and battling with exhaustion or the fibromyalgia pain I experienced day and night.

CHAPTER SIX

Guardian Angel, Kimberly

Back to when I walked through the door of the house trailer, Jo asked me right off if I wanted to rent the place for she had found a teaching job somewhere else. Not too long after I moved in was when my friend Kimberly came into my life. In the second visit, she asked "who works on you?" I said, "my eldest daughter-in-law helps me." Although I'm concerned about being a burden. To make a long story short, Kimberly asked me what to do and to teach her how to do the treatments that I needed. After that, she would stop in as much as our schedules allowed. She lived down the road just a couple of miles, which worked out great for she didn't have to go out of her way to stop in.

During this time of just meeting Kimberly, my health was going even further south, due to the added stress in my life, and no time in which to have the time to take for the extra rest my body required. So in the following few months, there was like five or six times, I knew I wasn't going to wake up the next morning, so guess who stopped in, telling me she was supposed to work on me, Kimberly!!! I never called or let her know how I was feeling! What else is strange is that I wasn't ever scared or even thought to call my kids or anyone for that matter, it was kind of like when I saw the angel on my front bumper of my car when I had the wreck. It never even occurred to me that I should be worried or concerned for my well being. So I'd say the Lord was obviously stepping in!

You may be asking yourself by now why I never went to the doctor. Well, I did see two different doctors. One diagnosed me as being too stressed, and the other doctor in a matter of fact attitude informed me it was all in my head. And those diagnoses were determined after all the testing they did for me.

This was approximately thirty years ago. At that time, my energy and pain was continuing to worsen to the point of no return. I was taking two to three hour naps a day just to survive. With having two growing sons with no one to help in any way with everyday chores, it made things extremely difficult, to say the least.

Long story short, when my sons where almost high school aged, we found a medical doctor / alternative care doctor / acupuncturist in Las Vegas who saw people from all over the world. When he finished with the tests he ran on me, which also included a test on my energy level, he turned to me and asked, "Why are you still alive?" Well, I knew exactly what he was talking about, for I felt as though someone unplugged my battery. Surprisingly enough, I didn't die!

I replied, "I have no idea!" Thinking back, if I had known some of what I have learned since I've taken some of my classes, my reply would have been, "Why, Doctor! You must have at least a little energy to die. And since I have none, I am still here!"

CHAPTER SEVEN

The Culprit

Recollecting back approximately ten years from around this time, was the second time I escaped death which resulted from developing severe toxemia during my pregnancy with my eldest son which consequently triggered the weakening of my body's immune system that prepared my body for the full onslaught of Lyme disease after he was born. I didn't realize what I was dealing with till years later. And as a result of the weakening of my body's immune system, the toxemia had triggered I realize now it was preparing my body for the ravaging of West Nile disease to attack as well years later. I've never had the ability or the right tools (bodywork) and protocols to recuperate from these diseases until I discovered the Body Code and Systemic Formulas in the last couple of years. I can now look back at how the Lord was directing my path to have meant the people who have entered into my life who helped guide me down my path to the doors of opportunities to open for learning how to help not only myself but also others as well who suffer from Lyme and West Nile. I was, let's say in a very unstable marriage.

I called my mom to see if I could come home with my two awesome baby sons. Well, let's just say my mom was not the most lovable person alive. To just give you another hint of how she was, she did disown me in her will, in which I can now see that the Lord made use of her annihilating me as a means, to direct me to the path I was to follow. I must say I am truly grateful my dad was a very special person who was loved by everyone that knew him. They farmed in northwest Missouri. Being a farmer, you would think she would be sure to get her two small grandsons and her daughter out of a bad situation and harm's way? As you guessed she did say, "No! You are married and left home and the Catholic church, so you are on your own now." Yes, at the time, that was a very hard thing to swallow! As I look back now, by moving back there I would have never gotten any help with my illness, let alone had the opportunities to learn the things I have.

So after my sons were raised, I did leave and once again long story short, I acquired a wonderful little corn dog shop called Cowpokes in the mall in Chubbuck, Idaho. In the first two weeks of getting my shop, I had an invention I wanted to put on the market. I had an appointment in Salt Lake with a company to see what I needed to do. This is where the Lord put his toe in or actually his whole foot in the door!

On the drive down, I started having one of those sleepy spells, so I pulled off the interstate to grab something to eat and drink. When I got back into the car and approached the freeway, I felt like my brother Charlie (who had passed away with a brain tumor approximately three years before) was with me in the car. Tears started to run, then I felt like someone was in my back seat, in the passenger seat, as well as someone sitting behind me and at that time, there wasn't even a piece of lint back there. The feeling was so strong, I almost just pulled over to take a look in the trunk. So instead of pulling over to check the trunk, I just kept going then an hour later, traffic was stopped on the freeway due to workmen painting the lines on the freeway. Right before coming to a full stop, I noticed there was a huge angel hovering on my right front bumper, seeing the angel was as normal as if a friend was in the car with me. I also had the feeling not to pull up too close to the van in front of me as I was coming to a complete stop. Then I heard the squealing tires, knowing full well someone was going to get slammed big-time! I looked around and noticed the lanes on both sides of me had backed up traffic, so with that I knew, yep, it was me! I got smacked while at a dead stop sixty-five mph! Never hitting the steering wheel or breaking anything not even hitting my head in the windshield! Which I do remember being up and over the steering wheel.

Time seemed to stop, so I had a quick conversation with the Lord, which went like this, "Lord, if I can walk out of this, I won't complain about my pain." The ambulance driver got in the car with me, I told him I didn't need the ambulance for some reason. I just knew he could check out my knee that got smashed into the dash, it was feeling like it had shattered. He checked it out for me and said it didn't feel broken or out of place. Later, I did have x-ray and an MRI to be on the safe side. I had long hair all one length down to my elbows at that time. The one thing that surprised me the most was where I found my strong metal hair clips, that I used to pull and hold the strands of hair, on the sides of my head up. When I found them, they were just barely hanging at the ends of my hair! I also acquired a pretty good whiplash out of it as well. Now I ask you, how's that for doing what you want to do with your life? Keep reading, there's more plans I had for my life, that you will see as you continue to read. :)

I had that little corndog shop for three years or I should say, the Lord allowed me to have it for three years, for that is exactly how I feel about it. Due to the fact I was still very ill, I had always wanted or at least a little cute bakeshop to make my homemade cinnamon rolls and bread, pies, etcetera. Since I was still at least able to be vertical, I prayed and said to the Lord, "Lord, you know how I feel and just how much Tylenol I'm going to have to take every day to even just get by, so I know, Lord, you will make it so that I can have and run this little shop myself or you will take me home." (I had to take so much over the counter pain medication that I should have gone into liver failure in a few months!) So He did just that three years later after I more than doubled the revenue coming in the very first year I had it! I was planning on keeping it forever and passing it on to my kids. I did so love my shop and the people that stopped by for my corn dogs and, yes, there are not words to express how much I still miss it. You may be wondering what happened to it. Well, the mall sold. If you go there now, you will see for yourself the halls are empty. I hung on as long as I could. I had even had an old bread van converted into corn dog van and set it up down in Old Town, just off

Main Street. I was able to run it most of the summer of 2004. What happened next was diffidently definitely not expected!

The city decided to redo some of the plumbing under the streets! So I stayed once again as long as I could. When the day came that I could no longer get my van in and out, I walked out to the sidewalk looked around to see if there was a place to park my van that I hadn't seen yet. Of course, there was nothing. So since I had nowhere to go, I just looked up to heaven (knowing full well someone would call the people in the white coats to take me away!) So with that, I totally understand how a person feels when they lose everything for at that moment, reality sat in big-time! I said, "Okay, Lord, I am going to the health food store where I frequently shop at to see if the poster ad for massage classes was still there." And amazingly enough, it was still there, so I immediately called. The instructor answered, I asked about classes, and he told me he was starting his next class in two weeks! So once again, long story short, here I am now, taking the best supplements made "in my book," and this is why I can say this is.

If you have noticed that I mentioned I've been to and working with different doctors, and taking different brand of supplements, there just hasn't been anything that has helped me like Systemic Formula's product has. You may be asking, in what ways have they helped so much? Well, remember when I mentioned how tired I was? I am listing a few things I have battled with. One of the very worst is when I drive for six to nine hours to Wyoming, where my office is located. When I would pull over to take a nap, my chest area would hurt so, with also sensations of pressure. I also felt though I had been given a drug, for my head would feel so groggy, to the point that I would feel as though I was going into spasms or convulsions and then die! And yes, I've asked doctors about that issue as well but no one can pinpoint it. Not even a EKG or other heart testing. It was getting to the point right before I started taking these supplements that I was going to have to stop traveling to Wyoming to work. As you have most likely figured out, I don't know when to stop.

Then there's the 9:00 to 11:00 spell I have or, I should say, had every morning! When I felt like I just needed to sit down and croak (or die) being the same thing! Yes, every morning like clockwork, and yes, it happened while at work as well. I was finding that according to the Horary Clock it was spleen time. As I kept searching for answers over time, I found the cause of these episodes was my colon that was causing this upset every morning.

Before I discovered the source of all the episodes was my colon, I would take supplements that were for boosting energy. I found they would at least get me through, in order to stay vertical and go through the motions and all else I needed to do in a day's work.

Well, you guessed it, the Systemic Formulas supplements that I took, which I determined what my body needed through the Body Code method of muscle testing. I still cannot believe it that I'm healed up from those horrific episodes as well! Remember how it was impossible for me to fast and impossible to lose weight? I am now able to do those things and in only just a month being on the supplements! I'm also not feeling like I need a two- to three-hour nap in the afternoons! Amazing! Only those of you who have or are going through any type of illness that afflicts and is debilitating to your quality of life can relate to what I am talking about.

Below, you will find the list of supplements I tested for in conjunction of using the Body Code work to begin the rest of my healing process.

How I came across Systemic Formulas was through the Body Code program course that I took on line to become a certified practitioner, due to having Body Code treatments for a year, then after falling and breaking my wrist, I decided to take the Body Code Class. If I hadn't had a broken wrist, I most likely would have never found the time to do it, for it was quite time consuming! ***So amazingly enough, that is how I found out about the Systemic Formulas products!*** Wouldn't ya say I had a bit of direction (to say the least) coming from the good Lord above? Amen.

CHAPTER EIGHT

The "Supplement Yo-Yo Effect"

This is the list of supplements that my body tested for first, using the Body Code muscle testing technique.

- Systemic Formula's 5 Chinese Element Earth Sedate: this helps to keep my energy in balance). As I have mentioned before, through my experience with a person's journey to healing is to bring their energy into balance. Then from there, retrain it to become stable. This is where the Chinese elements come into play, for I am finding that they do it all! That is, they not only bring the energy into balance, but also keep it in balance as well.
- Systemic Formula's Gf Thyroid: Gf Thyroid builds and balances the thyroid gland. This formula supports the thyroid gland's role as a master control gland in producing normal, healthy metabolism. Gf assists the major metabolic actions of the endocrine systems. Helpful in supporting a healthy weight and in combating jet lag.
- Systemic Formula's Builder 2: Designed to be paired with a BioFunction formula that targets a specific tissue (e.g., B [Brain] + no. 2 [Builder] in tandem). This formula provides nutritional support for cellular integrity of the targeted tissue or organ during its normal building cycle. Helps relax the targeted tissue and enhance its self-maintenance processes during the tissue's restful, reconstruction cycle.

- o It supports the tissues' inherent building function during the building cycle.
- o It's great for rebuilding (e.g., postexercise, postcleansing, etcetera).
- o It increases impact of BioFunction formulas.
- Systemic Formula's Metabo-Shake (vanilla and chocolate): I tested well for both. The vanilla Metabo-Shake is a highly potent metabolic formula, which provides a pure macro and micro nutrient profile. Our formula is specifically designed to support patients struggling with poor diet. Using Metabo-Shake along with a balanced diet and moderate physical activity promotes a healthy metabolism, supports the pancreas sugar balance and optimal cardiovascular functions. Metabo Shake is also a good source of potassium. Diets containing foods that are a good source of potassium and that are low in sodium may reduce the risk of high blood pressure and stroke.
- Systemic Formula's Glycemic Synulin: it supplies botanical nutrients from all over the world plus a patented chromium chelate for normal, healthy cell membrane and mitochondrial uptake of glucose for production of ATP (Adenosine Triphosphate)—the chemical energy of life. Based on HerbalomicTM research, the botanical ingredients are selected as nourishment for the epigenetic metabolic functions of the citric acid and beta oxidation cycles. Supports whole body health via cellular energy nutrition. 4OH-Chromium-Isoleucinate contains a bioavailable source of chromium and isoleucine, which assists insulin in the biochemical regulation of fat, carbohydrate, and protein metabolism.
  - * *Chromium and Isoleucine may support insulin-mediated glucose uptake by cells.*
  - * *Assists insulin in the biochemical regulation of fat, carbohydrate, and protein metabolism.*
- Systemic Formula's Neurosyn: neurosyn is formulated to support healthy brain aging, cognition, and memory by

beneficially modulating the metabolism of the neurotransmitter acetylcholine and providing neuroprotection. This advanced formula features clinically effective levels of the Sulbutiamine form of B1, huperzine A (HUPA), Alpha GPC, Acetyl L-Carnitine, phosphatidylserine and a proprietary herbalomic blend for multidimensional support for neurological health. Research suggests that Sulbutiamine and HUPA may be able to cross the blood-brain barrier to beneficially influence acetylcholine metabolism and provide antioxidant protection. In addition, laboratory studies on epigallocatechin-3-gallate (EGCG) antioxidant and DNA protective properties, suggesting it may have beneficial effects on brain aging.

  * *Preliminary controlled studies suggest that Noopept may enhance inhibitory synaptic transmission in the hippocampus, which is the proposed mechanism of action for memory support. Supportive but not conclusive research demonstrates the ability of Alpha-GPC to rapidly deliver choline to the brain across the blood-brain barrier and act as a biosynthetic precursor of the acetylcholine neurotransmitter.*

- Systemic Formula's Eventa (cellular enzyme corrector): eventa supports optimal cellular function of the many Nitric Oxide Synthase (NOS) pathways. Proper NOS management is critical to lowering oxidative stress on the cells' organelles and maintaining efficient cellular metabolic functions. It provides amino acids, nutrients, and phytonutrients that can help build the cellular enzyme systems that support muscle integrity, organ and gland health, and increased energy. Eventa is part of the family of Systemic Formulas' Cellular Healing research. Often Used post Exercise or in times when optimal nutrient blood flow is critical.

- Systemic Formula's Collagen ECM formula. Collagen is the predominant form of protein throughout the body. It's part of connective tissues, bones, cartilage, and supports red blood cells and tissue integrity. With aging, the body's production of collagen decreases, which results in many health issues. Supplementing with collagen boosts the body's metabolic processes and can help offset the decline in collagen due to aging. Collagen proteins are long chain amino acid structures, particularly rich in glycine, which supports metabolic functions and detoxification. Collagen plays a vital role in joint maintenance and the body's normal joint health processes. It also is essential for skin elasticity (Collagen Type I) and thus has gained a reputation for skin, hair, and nail normal health and youthfulness. Collagen is particularly beneficial to the skin's dermis (the deep layer) health, especially for people over age fifty. Collagen has the amazing ability to support muscle, bone, and connective tissue in balance with body fat, thus supporting a favorable muscle mass and body composition. Eggshell membranes are powerhouses of nutrients similar to Collagen types I and V. They are rich in glucosamine sulfate, chondroitin sulfate, hyaluronic acid, glycosaminoglycans and amino acids—all vital nutrients for joint health and strong connective tissues throughout the body. The availability of these supportive amino acid chains provides the body the specific molecules it requires to maintain overall integrity of his structure and functionality.

Hyaluronic acid: supports the body's innate collagen synthesis processes, i.e. the body's inherent youthful cell maintenance processes.

Collagen ECM is the world's most potent and complete formula containing:
- o   Type I: Skin, tendons, vascular ligatures, bones, and organs
- o   Type II: Cartilage
- o   Type III: Reticulate fibers (forms crosslinks for connective tissue strength and durability)

- o Type IV: Basement membrane strength (the extra cellular matrix and skin support)
- o Type V: Supports hair health, placenta integrity, and cell structure strength
- o Type X: Supports articular cartilage

- Systemic Formula's Vitamin Detox: high potency, broad-spectrum detoxifier; an excellent drainage formula for use in any cleansing, elimination program, and/or detoxification program, especially for organ detoxification. In addition, support is provided for the liver, especially the left lobe, and the kidneys. Helps avoid cleansing reactions (Herxheimer's).

These next two heart supplements, I tested for about a week after I started taking the supplements above. Within three days of taking them I drove to Wyoming to my office there, I had energy and endurance all the way except for the last twenty miles! And I have not experienced those spells since, that I mentioned before, where I had to pull over to take nap, and having the spells where my chest became tight, and didn't know whether I was going to go into convulsions or something.

Then on my way back home to Idaho, I never experienced anything of the spells at all!

Now that's AMAZING!

- Systemic Formula's Heart Cardiovascular provides nutritional tissue support for the arteries, veins, and capillaries. Ingredients in the formula were used ethnobotanically as a mild lymphatic cleanser for "cleanup" of the body's "red and white" blood systems. This formula supports a healthy circulation and blood pathway integrity.
- Systemic Formula's Heart Energy formula feeds the heart by providing a host of natural ingredients—vitamins, minerals, enzymes, amino acids, essential fatty acids—plus herbs for a total support approach to the heart's energy. The latest research on optimal heart health leads directly to

the heart cells' mitochondria and their ability to maintain optimal energy for the heart muscle. This comprehensive formula addresses the multifacets of heart energy support. It provides nutrients used in: Creating and maintaining sustained energy optimal production of ATP optimal cardiac function.

- Systematic Formula: RPM, In the 21st Century, many people suffer from chronic immunological inflammation, (cited by Time Magazine, 2/2004 as the "silent killer")—a condition where the body's innate immune system works overtime compared to its adaptive immune system. Science has identified that certain polyunsaturated (PUFA) molecules called EPA and DHA are required to provide active metabolites—Resolvins, Protectins, Maresins—used when the body determines that the initiating phase of inflammation is fulfilled and the Resolution Phase can begin. Thus, inflammation does not simply vanish, it must first actively resolve. Scientific research points to the fact that the humandiet requires more pro-resolving molecules to keep up with the demands of the current environment. RPM Omega is formulated to provide the body nutritional EPA/DHA, plus synergetic White Willow Extract to support the resolving phase of the natural inflammation activities.

After being on the above supplements for a month, I found that I started muscle testing for detox supplements, such as the Accell. It seemed that my body needed nutrients that it could absorb and utilize to become stronger as well stabilizing my energy before my body began testing positive for detoxing products. This I did not find surprising that my body did not test for the detoxification programs first due to the fact, as those of us who have done detox programs we all know it takes energy when we put our bodies through a detoxification program. I tested the supplements, along with the Accell, to see if I still needed to continue to take all the supplements that I first tested for. This proved I needed to cut out some of the supplements for a short time while detoxing and some of those were the heart ones and even the Chinese formulas! Due to the fact my energy was actually holding stable on it's own, I might add! I am continuing to grow stronger and building more endurance than ever.

I find it very important to muscle test a formula with the ones you are already taking to see if it is too much for your body or if you need to cut one out so you don't overload your system. For even though all those supplements were very good for me, when my body test for something else, I have found it just does not need everything you can throw at it. I've seen this a lot in my practice, people will bring all their supplements and herbs that they are taking for me to muscle test for them. I find most times they are just overloading their systems.

This is another reason why I am writing this book so that people will be cautioned about this very thing. It is so easy to overload your system due to all the media and ads out there claiming this and that, and people are so desperate to feel better, they find their vitamin cabinets are overloaded as well and then in turn become overwhelmed, which causes huge disappointments because they are still not getting a whole lot better or stopped completely improving. That's when they find themselves taking a few things for a while then read about another product then buy that one because they know this one has to be "the one!" I call this the *"supplement yo-yo" effect*, which is a hard thing for me to admit to. I as well, have been guilty of doing this very thing for years! Which in effect I did start to feel better at first, then as time went on I found I stopped improving and once again started to decline. I have been playing with the *supplement yo-yo* for approximately forty years, 'til I started taking Systemic Formula's products. By staying on these products, I find my endurance continuing to build as long as I do not indulge in food additives, which causes me huge setbacks.

As my health progresses, I find my endurance has exceeded over and above what I ever expected it could become. Even now, I still continue to muscle test myself to see if I need to change to a different formula after I've finish up a supplement or to see if I need to cut something out of my program or to cut my dosage on a product as I continue to heal.

CHAPTER NINE

Lesson to be Learned About Eating Wrong Foods

This is my answer to a question of a client about having a possible relapse of Lyme disease and/or stressed out.

"Yes, in my experience, you can do too much of the wrong foods. It seems the Lyme will go into remission off and on 'til you get it totally cleared and stabilize your energy levels. I see people have setbacks or symptoms of Lyme and West Nile due to breaking their healthy diet, including myself! Like when I was in Wyoming a while back, I didn't have time to make meals. I ate a piece of a popular carryout or take home and bake pizza every day for three days! After that third day, I was heading back to Idaho the following morning. On awaking, I found my neck had a horrible kink in it. I don't like to admit it, although, I must say, I was in trouble! So my son and daughter-in-law. Worked on it enough so that I could continue my journey back home to Idaho. I also used essential oils with a hot towel. About three hours later, I was able to drive. I had to get on the road due to snowstorms coming in, I had three passes to go over, and they aren't pretty or safe during a snow storm. I've been ill ever since. I've been back for a week now. My neck is much better, but I still feel ill and not much endurance. I thought I was strong enough by then that I could handle the take home and bake yourself pizza! Still learning."

One thing I have noticed is how Lyme and West Nile, especially West Nile seems to create extreme food sensitivities and especially to food additives. And a person needs to remember as mentioned before, it takes energy to heal so when we ingest these food additives (like food colorings) that can cause muscle pain as well as other symptoms. MSG, which is an abbreviation for monosodium glutamate, can cause migraines, brain fogginess, mood changes, and can make one unable to focus or function well in their life, I am discovering that these symptoms can last from two weeks and even up to thirty days. Not only do I find these symptoms producing mayhem within myself, but other people as well have told me they too have realized they are suffering from "food additive trauma." I am continuing to find these extreme sensitivities in the Lyme and West Nile victims.

Just as I ate the pizza, I felt disabled brain-wise (*those of you who have experienced brain fog know what I mean about your brain feeling disabled*) as well as physical pain for about a week! And the result of this is realizing *that **I'm still learning*** just how temperamental ingesting food additives can be to my life! People would often express to me about how difficult it is to know what to eat, they often ask me. "What do you eat?" My comeback is nothing prepared, no mixes, nothing with food colorings, or that says "natural food flavorings" (this can act as an umbrella for MSG, so be careful about this one on labels). And as for using herbs and spices in my cooking, if it has listed in the ingredients label anything other than herbs and spices, I won't buy it. I also wanted to add here about my experience with potatoes (not sweet potatoes) I have found they cause my first joints in my finger to swell and also causes my index finger to bend towards my middle finger. I found these results through Body Code when I started to test for any possible allergens in the family of night shade vegetables.

After I cut out the potatoes from my diet, my fingers have gotten straighter and the inflammation has gone out of the joints.

I must admit this was a hard thing to do for potatoes are one of my favorite foods next to chocolate. Especially my homemade twice baked potatoes that I add freshly graded Nutmeg to, (*and you can't cheat by using store bought ground nutmeg for it doesn't work...sorry*) homemade Tiramisu and my homemade flour-less chocolate cake with a spoon full or two…of "made from scratch" chocolate pudding *(to which I owe my good friend Kassia who decided to try out the combination during a day of baking some of our favorite things.)* And then you must add a couple of large dollops of homemade whipped cream on top, to which I add powered sugar to it, so it will stay holding it's shape the next day.

I also have found that while I was in such despair with West Nile, I craved pizza and potato chips! So when a client would come in my door who was suffering from, or I suspected they might be suffering from Lyme or West Nile, the first thing I ask is "do you by any chance have cravings for pizza and potato chips" the answer…as you guessed, it is always a definite…YES! It never ceases to amaze me!

And then I check the feet to see if there are any till tale signs of parasite infection, then the next question I ask is "out of curiosity, do you crave ice cream?" And once again this is always a definite…YES!

Through most of my years of practice after I started putting all the indications of West Nile together that I have seen, one of the major signs happens to be very dry skin that also can have a thick texture and feels a bit like elephant skin to me in the affected areas of the figures, hands, feet, or all of these areas could be affected all at once. I've noticed even when I apply lotion the skin continues to stay dry and continues to have the thick texture to it. And the amazing thing is…once the person starts to heal from the West Nile the skin also heals becoming subtle once again!

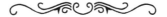

Below is a persons left foot that may show signs of parasite infection, where the arrows are pointing to deep lines that may indicate scarring from the parasites, the brown arrow shows the puffiness that also may indicate inflammation in the tissues, these are some of the most common signs I look for. As you see I marked the locations of the areas of bladder, ureter tube, kidney, sigmoid colon, stomach and lungs to give you an idea of what those of us that do reflexology check to see if there are any puffiness or tightness in the muscle tissues and also anything unusual on the skin. Those of you who are not familiar with reflexology, the sigmoid colon area lies on the left foot only, just as it is in the body. For when you put the feet side by side it becomes a map of the whole body. So from the way these areas are looking with the lines and puffiness going on, this person may be having most of their health issues in these areas. Sometimes these lines vary and can look as though they are bleeding. Whenever I've seen those types of lines on peoples feet, it can be a sign those people have been suffering for a very long time with their health issues. What I have noticed through my years of practice are how these lines soften up, the redness disappears and they "V" out into softer lines after a person goes on a parasite protocol.

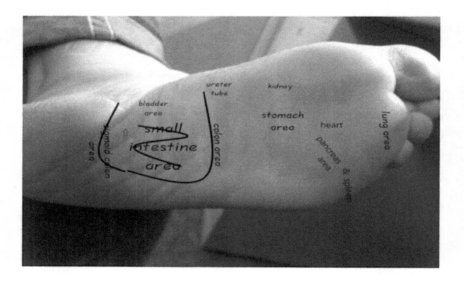

Also notice the puffiness around the big toe and at the base of the big toe which is the neck area, notice how the skin on the toe and heel appears to be dry and flaky as well. I've also seen these types of issues disappear with a parasite protocol treatment.

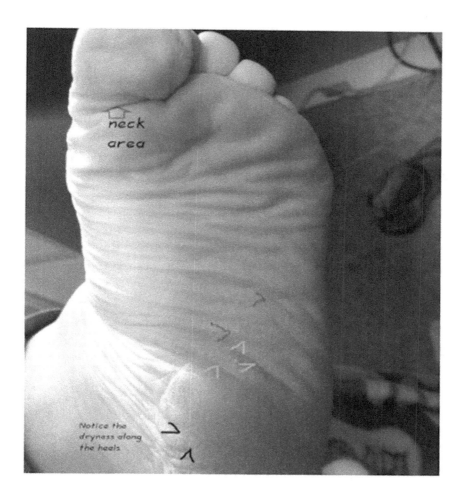

In the photo above notice the puffiness around the red arrows, for these too will also soften up and disappear along with the dryness you see along the heel.

These tell tale signs are an indication to me that this person is not feeling so well and most likely has not felt well for some time. After examining her feet I asked how her energy and over all general health is doing, she said "not so good" come to find out she is dealing with cyst growing on her kidneys that she inherited from her mother. It is such an amazing thing to see how the body can heal when given the correct treatments.

As studies show a person can inherit parasitic infections.

I must say I've found that not all parasite formulas coincide. I have seen the most effective results of ridding the body of parasites after my clients and including myself have taken the Systemic Formulas's parasite formulas. In which I use the Body Code to muscle test for each person's individual needs, for instance, which formula their body needs first in priority and then how many (a day which may also include a certain time of day) and how many bottles they may need to take to overcome a particular type of parasite infection. I also do a Body Code treatment to get an understanding of and to find out the reasons and/or causes why the person contacted the parasite infection in the first place and then clear those findings to allow the energies and circulation to flow better through the body which creates as we all know, a more efficient healing to take place, then from here I can work on clearing the parasitic frequencies. This is why I am so grateful for the Body Code! I do these types of Body Code treatments for myself, this is my secret of how I'm continuing to help myself progress to a better state of health than I was in before I became certified in the Body Code and finding Systemic Formulas products.

I find by preparing all my own food, I heal much faster as well as continuing to have those wonderful days of having a clear mind and to be able to function well on my life's journey. And I love that feeling! When I have those times of messing that up, it's very disheartening for me! But during those times, I feel the good Lord uses this lesson to prove to myself, as well as to share with others just how extremely disabling these food additives are to those of us who are food sensitive whether it is due to West Nile, Lyme, or just having allergens to certain foods for whatever reasons.

People ask me what I eat, what makes me feel the best, and have the most energy I find is eating salad that is made of fresh and spinach, kale, and chard, then sometimes I'll throw in other fresh vegetables like fresh mushrooms, or sliced zucchini and cucumbers, cabbage, cauliflower, broccoli, carrots, and bean sprouts, then I mix this with the spinach, chard, and kale salad. I love a bit of feta cheese or goat cheese over it along with some sunflower seeds, a bit of dried cranberries, or dried blueberries and some boiled eggs. Then I like to mix my dressings by drizzling some homemade ranch dressing along with some homemade poppy seed dressing. If I don't have the time to do that then I'll purchase ones that are MSG-free.

I've gotten away from eating any lettuce of any kind. I find it is harder for me to digest and besides that I just don't feel as well, if I do eat any at all I find it I'm okay with Romaine lettuce. Recently I have added Systemic Formulas #619 Ketabo-Vanilla Shake to my diet. I have noticed even more energy. It also is helping my cravings. Plus it helps that it tastes like a desert drink. And feeling even better since I have started watching my carb intake.

Ketabo-Shake provides highest-quality, core-level, broad-range, ingredient-expansive nutrition for people who want to boost their dietary diversity while adhering meticulously to the macro-nutrients that support ketogenesis—the production of ketones (acetoacetate, beta-hydroxybutyrate, and acetone) from fatty acids that serve the body for abundant brain energy and cellular fat-burning for mito-chondrial-produced energy.

Cholesterol 38 mg, Sodium 169 mg, Total Carbohydrate 7.5 g, Dietary Fiber 1 g, Total Sugars 1 g Protein 12.7 g. You can find more information on my website including the #617—EXTRACELLULAR KETONES—BHB KETONES

As far as bread is concerned, I purchase sprouted breads. For pancakes (which I have once in a great while), I use almond flour but with a twist: I add extra eggs in the batter along with a bit of real vanilla flavoring, and a bit of mace spice. The addition of extra eggs not only provides you with extra protein but also keeps the pancakes from falling apart on me when I turn them over on the griddle. I must say, these almond flour pancakes surprised me with a lot of energy and stamina throughout the day. And as for my French toast, I use the sprouted grain bread so between the pancakes and my homemade French toast, they keep me from craving extra sweets that I love so much. One of my passions in life happens to be cooking and especially baking. So yes, it is hard not to eat all the extras like going out to eat at my favorite restaurants. Then on the flip side of the coin, it feels good to feel good! So when I stop and think about my favorite places to eat and then how it makes me feel afterwards, it's not worth it!

And as far as baked goods goes, my favorite is my homemade pies, for which I use honey for sweetening. My goal is to find time in the future to write a cookbook that has recipes of some of my favorite foods to share with you. So keep your eyes peeled!

Things I've Noticed that May Cause Back Pain

I also wanted to add something to this chapter that through my practice as a licensed massage therapist and certified Body Code practitioner, I have noticed that while working on peoples backs, who drink sodas, sports drinks, too much beer, (some brands I find cause more low back and sciatic pain than others) hard liqueur and whiskys (I find is the very worst of liqueurs) black tea, and even green tea, (I have found green tea to tighten up ribs T-8 through T-11. I find this with the people who are eating a healthy diet and that due to media they are lead to believe it is ok to ingest large quantities) *ice water and ice drinks of any kind hardens up their rib cage to the point that the ribs are not flexible at all! To the degree of loosing the ribs flexability, of course depends on how much of these substances are in their diet.* Which makes their ribs feel like brittle wood, and their rib cage is not flexible as it should be. These people also come in complaining of back pain. So by going off these substances in conjunction with treatments, which also include lymphatic drain and giving time for their ribs to heal, they become flexible once again. I would like to conclude here that I have found the substances listed above can also cause inflammation in the sciatic nerve, not only that, it can cause havoc with the colon as well which in-turn can create immense discomfort in the left hip which I am sure many of you have unfortunately, experienced.

Also if one is suffering from Lyme or West Nile, the lymphatics also seem to have difficulty draining in the left hip as well, which can cause even more pressure on the nerves and creating even more pain in that left hip area. Well, don't feel too bad, for I never thought about how the body operates either, until I started studying more on how our digestive system functions. And I must say everyone who has been in my office with complaints about their stomach upsets along with other digestive issues also uses ice in their drinks and/or uses the refrigerator's water dispenser or stashes all their bottled water and other beverages in the frig so they'll be nice and cold, and they also use their microwave…*so "they can make sure to consume the daily recommended requirement of radiated food substances"…I say this to get you to think about what you're doing to your digestion…Question…Is it okay to consume a bit of toxic waste every day and not expect the digestion to retaliate over time? I find these are some of the reasons why my clients are in the age group of mid-forties and up due to their digestion's are starting to retaliate. Here is an example: I had someone awhile back come in to see me who was not feeling well at all this person happens to be in the mid-sixties who's main complaint was when she had to visit the bathroom she'd have only a moments notice to make it there in time! (I will not highlight on the reason why, for I'm sure you can imagine…) She also informed me that she had been to see many doctors and thousands of dollars later, **and not only that she's been battling with these issues for twenty years!!!** And, she still hasn't found the reasons for her issues. After listening to her story, I decided to take a look at her feet (which was showing indications of a parasitic infection.) After I shared with her what her feet where telling me, I then started to check for tightness in her abdominal area, the first thing I came across was her solar plex area which was very tight and very uncomfortable to the touch, so as I just rested my hand there to help the area to relax, I noticed it felt…I will say… "on the rubbery side of things!" I know this will sound a bit strange to you…but here goes anyway…her energy field said one word to me… and that word was "Microwave." So I shared that information of what her energy field revealed to me. Her response was "Why YES! I use the Microwave EVERY DAY! Because I do not like to cook and plus I don't have the time!" So after doing a treatment for her to help the organs drain* *more efficiently, the solar plex area had drained a lot allowing the tension in the muscles to dissipate…which put her in a much more relaxed state, and she was beginning to feel much better overall. I also found that her organ drain-lobe areas were also very tight to the point that I could not even press in on her abs!!! It's no wonder she was at her wits end when she walked in my door. Her energy looked to me…as though she was twisted in every direction and, then scrunched! The ending of this story is…she gave me a big hug of appreciation and walked out the door not only taller but, with an elevated mood and, a big smile on her face with confidence of having found a path to a healthier life. Amen!…*

It's amazing to watch those people with stomach and digestion complaints start feeling much better when they do nothing more than give up the cold drinks and replace them with room temperature water (which I will add fresh squeezed lemon or lime juice laced with a bit of honey) and drinking something hot (after a meal) like herbal teas such as peppermint or chamomile which is known to quite good for digestions, or even just a cup of warm water after eating will help that scrumptious homemade butter melt more efficiently and also allowing the digestive muscles do their job without having to work super hard due to the *ice storm* they experience every time you eat. Then with some abdominal bodywork *(massage)* to help open the organs' drain lobes and coax the organs to drain *(as we all know when debris backs up in our organs then it becomes toxic allowing disease to set in.)* For those of you not so familiar with how the digestion works, the hair like fibers *(villi & microvilli)* in the small intestine picks up the nutrition from the food and liquids we ingest then sends it out to feed our body through the nervous system and yes including our limbs, hands, fingers and even our toes to help relax all muscle spasms in the digestion areas which also allows me to massage the stomach down out of the ribs and diaphragm and then do some reflexology for them, they soon start to feel much better, and as long as they have nothing else medical wise going on, and when they report back to me they tell me their acid reflux issues have gone away.

As many of you have heard and know the feet have areas that correlate with every area in the body. The digestion areas in the feet happen to lay on the bottom, of the feet, therefore the foods we consume could be the cause for creating discomfort in a persons feet. Please understand here as I mentioned before that when we are under stress from illness or life in general we can be more sensitive to even "healthy foods" till we can get ourselves back into balance. So when someone comes in to see me about their pain in their feet, I always ask first off, how their diet is, and do some muscle testing for them in conjunction with a Body Code treatment to see if they have any inherited allergens and/or trapped emotions, or other issues that may be causing the allergens. If allergens do show up, by doing a Body Code treatment for them their allergens may clear up.

Now then in this next bit of information, I strongly suggest you see your health care provider to rule out any underlying health issues, and ***do not attempt to do a treatment on yourself, due to other steps that need to be taken first.*** Which I will teach in my Nerve Tissue Release Technique classes, I mention later on in chapter twelve.

**Tip: No time to cook? How about putting your dinner in a crockpot, you can even take it with you to work and plug it in so you can keep an eye on it…if that's not an option they do have timers on some of them to shut off automatically. If you get tired of the crockpot… use it as an oven by putting your food into a baking dish and sitting on a rack in the crockpot, then turn the temperature up to your normal settings that you bake with. You can use an oven thermometer so you know when the crockpot reaches the desired temperature. Be sure not to take the lid off during cooking so it doesn't lose the heat.

To heat something up quick and have it taste much better than "heated up microwaved food"…if you don't have a griddle you can use a large skillet to warm your food up by using it as a griddle, so what you do is put a bit of water in the bottom just enough to get some steam going, then add your food to it, you can spread it out or cut it in smaller pieces so it will heat up faster. Then after you put your food in, put a lid over it that is smaller than the skillet… so it will fit down into the skillet covering the food. Then adjust the heat so as not to burn your dinner. Usually medium to medium-high heat will do the job. I believe you will be amazed at just how quick your dinner will heat up. This is how they warm things up in the restaurants and get your hamburgers cooked quicker. The trick is to not to add too much water so you won't have a watered-down meal. Just like with anything else do a practice run by warming up a small amount of something. If I'm warming up a chicken casserole instead of using water I'll use a bit of chicken broth. Same goes for anything with beef, I'll use a bit of beef broth rather than the water. I also use this process to warm up bread, I just use a lower temperature, and careful on the water! You even want to tip the lid a bit to allow some of the steam to escape so it won't come out soggy.

If someone has complaints about their digestion, especially bloating of the stomach, low energy, and then if I notice the slug-gishness of the lymphatic system, I will do a Body Code treatment to see how the spleen *(as well as the other organs that lie under the ribs)* is doing since it happens to be the *largest lymphatic organ* in the body. It helps white blood cells to proliferate and initiates the appropriate immune response when necessary. I have noticed during bodywork treatments my ribs had incredibly tender points along the edge of them, *(five on each side)* I found that when another therapist would palpate these points I noticed my liver, gallbladder, stomach pan-creas, and spleen areas would start to drain, which in turn resulted in feeling better and the tightness that was under the edge of my ribs began to dissipate! Over time and bodywork sessions the organs under my ribs have become soft which allows my therapist to very gently massage under my ribs and this allows my diaphragm to…let's say "breath easier" which in-turns helps my breathing when I go up a set of stairs, or run up a hill.

How I came across these findings was through the inspiration to help and the experience of working with people and asking about their diets and if they drank any of these substances and what brands. After listening to what their drinks consists of, I ask if they happen to drink ice water and if they have ice in any of their other drinks. If their answer is a yes, then I will say, "let's pretend you are going to make a cake in-which the recipe calls for melted butter." Then I ask what happens to melted butter if you put that melted butter in the refrigerator before you blend it into the cake batter. As you guessed, their response is always the same, "you cannot stir it into the batter due to it hardening up." My come back to that is "now I want you to imagine…jumping into a bathtub of ice water." And then I ask "what would your muscles do?" Then I begin to paint another picture by having them imagine eating something like a piece of homemade bread still hot right out of the oven with plenty of freshly churned butter that you liberally spread over it and of course we need to top that with homemade strawberry preserves accompanied by nothing less than your favorite beverage which of course you made sure when you put the ice in, that it was clear to the top of your favorite glass you where using, so as to keep your beverage good and cold. "Now then" I ask "what do you think is going to happen not only to the involuntary muscles in your digestive track, but I want you to think of one other thing, what do you think is going to happen to that wonderful hot bread and all that scrumptious, freshly homemade butter that has melted just right after you spread it ever so carefully over your bread as not to smoosh it…after all it did just come out of a hot oven?"

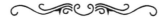

Dear Reader,

I believe you get the picture I just painted for you of what's going to happen with your digestive muscles and all the wonderful butter mingling with your favorite ice cold beverage in your stomach. Well don't feel too bad, for I never thought about it either before learning more of how our digestive system functions. And I must say everyone who has been in my office with complaints about their stomach upsets along with other digestive issues also uses ice in their drinks and/or uses the refrigerator's water dispenser or stashes all their bottled water and other beverages in the frig so they'll be nice and cold.

It's amazing to watch those people with stomach and digestion complaints start to feeling much better when they give up the cold drinks then with drinking something hot like herbal tea such as peppermint or chamomile which is known to quite good for digestions, or even just a cup of warm water after eating will help that scrumptious homemade butter melt more efficiently and also allowing the digestive muscles do their job without going through an ice storm every time you eat. Then with some abdominal bodywork *(massage)* and to help open the organs drain lobes and very gently massage to coax the organs to start draining, for as we all know when debris backs up in our organs then it becomes toxic overtime allowing disease to set in. For those of you not so familiar with how our digestion works, let's just say...long story short the hair like fibers *(villi & microvilli)* of the small intestine picks up the nutrition from the food and liquids we ingest then sends it out to the nervous system to feed our body, and yes including our limbs, hands, fingers and even our toes.

To help relax all muscle spasms in the digestion areas which also allows me to massage the stomach down out of the ribs and diaphragm and then do some reflexology for them, they soon start to feel much better, and as long as they have nothing else medical wise going on, for the most part they tell me their antacid issues went away. Next, I will share with you an easy simple exercise for you to do to help relax your stomach. First thing in the morning is to drink a tall glass of warm water give it a minute to help warm and relax the stomach muscles, then stand up on your tippy-toes and using your full weight then drop down on your heels. Do this four to six times. Then apply very light, gentle pressure with your finger tips of your right on the left ribs at the solar plex area just under the breast and then pull the tissues at the same time while applying the light pressure, and continue to pull very slowly over to the right rib. This may help to relax the sphincter muscle connecting the stomach and esophagus. (STOP! *If you have knee or ankle injuries. And also if you experience any pain by doing this exercise, visit your chiropractor or your health care provider to rule out any potential issues with your health.*) The warm water may help your stomach muscles relax allowing it to drop down from pressing up under the ribs into the diaphragm and to be able to re-position itself where it should be. That way it keeps food from backing up into the esophagus which may be the reason for creating one's heartburn. Then you should be able to run or walk up a hill or a set of stairs easier since there won't be as much pressure on the diaphragm. By drinking a glass of warm water first thing in the morning a half hour before eating or drinking anything else, may help rinse the debris from your colon easier, that the liver released into it in the middle of the night, plus your stomach, the small intestine, and the rest of your digestive tract may not have to work so hard due to not being in a frozen state from all the scrumptious icy cold drinks that tend to freeze up the muscle reflexes.

Enjoy to the fullest!
Kathy

**Note:* this is one of the techniques as well as how to help your organs drain more efficiently that I will go over with you in the classes that I will be offering for my Nerve Tissue Release Technique.*

I found it all to be very interesting that everyone through the last fifteen years has given me the same reports concerning their diets, unless of course, they've had some type of physical injury, that is cause to their pain, then that's a different story altogether.

By sharing these experiences, I'm hoping they will be an inspiration and an incentive to strengthen your willpower against adulterated foods.

CHAPTER ELEVEN

(SIBO) Small Intestinal Bacteria Overgrowth

***For more detailed information I have a video about SIBO to watch on my website.

SIBO…I wanted to mention just a bit about SIBO in my book since I have found a few people including a few therapists who have not heard of SIBO as to not overlook a possible issue with it on your healing journey. For more detailed information I have a video about SIBO to watch on my website. As research shows Lyme and West Nile may mutate into other diseases that I have seen happen. For instance West Nile mutating into spinal meningitis, therefore a person might want to see about being tested for West Nile. I've also seen people who were suffering from fibromyalgia who had actually contracted Lyme disease, including myself. This is why it is a good idea to work with someone qualified to help guide you in doing some sort of testing whether it's a blood test, muscle testing, or whatever your choice of a health care provider maybe.

Classic mistakes of SIBO…are not treating long enough. Mild: cases may be fixed in 7-14 days. Moderate: 4-6 weeks, as for Severe: cases can take up to three months on a protocol and in which case may need antibiotics. In which you will find more information in the next few pages.

Ileocecal Valve: when stuck open tends to allow colon matter to migrate into the small intestine.

SIBO…Classic Mistakes Some mistakes can include not addressing co-infections such as candida and parasites can be a reason for the recurrence of SIBO.

* Not treating long enough
* Mild cases may be fixed in 7-14 days
* Moderate 4-6 weeks
* *Severe cases can take up to 3 months on a protocol and may need antibiotics*

SIBO…Antibiotics

* **Rifaximin…**is a semi-synthetic antibiotic used for treating traveler's diarrhea and hepatic encephalopathy. It is derived from rifamycin, a naturally orccurring chemical produced by a bacterium called Streptomyces mediterranei.
* *Neomycin…*If constipation is an issue this may need to be added with Rifaximin

Probiotics-Lactobacilli can make worse in SIBO cases.

***Tips: Saccharomyces Cerevisiae Boulardii are great. In general spore or soil based seem to work best. Avoid fermented foods until fully recovered.*

Tips: products such as Tai-Ra-Chi and #4 VRM's may be added to your supplement protocol, which you can find on my website as well as in the supplement list in this book.

WO oil: This may be a massive help in ridding the body of these unwanted varmints. In which I have proven this works on a personal level.

As I had mentioned previously, years ago when I was in my late twenty's I went to two different doctors to see why I felt like I was dying due to being in so much pain and so exhausted all the time, after I went through all their testing one doctor told me "it was all in my head" the other doctor was more disciplined with his wording by informing me that I was just overly stressed! With that bit of news, I knew he was telling me that I was on my own to figure out why I felt so awful. So this is why after taking a class for research of live and dried blood *(microscopy work)* I purchased a scope to be able to keep a check on my healing progress and for others as well. I also must share this bit of news about my findings with the problem of totally relying on the scope for a health evaluation, is that I found my blood was improving and got to the point of looking very good, but then the problem was ***I still felt like I was dying*** and still no one could tell me why I was not feeling better! I also have taken peoples blood before working on them, and then I looked at their blood once again after their treatment to see if any changes actually took place in their blood during their bodywork treatment. I was curious about how much the bodywork treatment affected the blood.

I have done this very thing for a few of my friends who are clients of mine as well. And to my amazement...I will say this, I sold less supplements, when I would do their bodywork first and then look at their blood. Than I would have if I had done their blood work prior to the bodywork. I still am shocked at how much the blood changed after doing an hour treatment on people. After seeing these results I now understand even more of why I feel so much better after I figured out the right type of excising, bodywork treatments and nutrition programs I put together when I started doing Body Code for myself.

So, to just share with you what bodyworkers may experience with clients, lets say for example a client comes in that has discomfort in their low back, so when I begin their treatment I first work on their feet to see if any other areas are sore besides low back area, so, lets say kidney area is quite tender and puffy, I then ask how their kidneys treat them. If they say they haven't noticed anything different other than low back pain, I always suggest that they may want to check the situation out with their health care provider to cover all bases, in case of an underlying issue, which has happened a few times in my practice. Then, on the other hand, I've had a few people that have come to see me and not inform me about a particular issue, thinking it was of no importance. That's the reason why I am so grateful for the instructor I had due to making reflexology a requirement in his massage course. For now, I can joke with individuals who come to see me and especially if it's a person that is trying to hide just how they are really feeling, then I have to say to them…"you know you can not lie to a reflexologist!"

Below are symptoms that may be the cause of SIBO

*   Low stomach acid
*   Low digestive enzymes
*   Ileocecal valve (is sphincter muscle valve that separates the small intestine and the large intestine. Its function is to limit the reflux of colonic contents into the ileum. Approximately two liters of fluid enters the colon daily through the ileocecal valve.

The ileocecal valve is the only site in the gastrointestinal tract that is used for vitamin B-12 and bile acid absorption.

When the ileocecal valve is open this allows good bacteria from colon to migrate into the small intestine. This is why pressing in and massaging it in a clock wise motion twice and palpating it a few times can help it function better. But, of course you will not want to do this, but once a day unless you have a chronic issue and then a couple of times a day (you may also check with your chiropractor or alternative care physician to help you), then just check to see if the area feels tight morning and night. It's very important to never over stimulate!

Do to lymph nodes around the organ drain lobes I have found during a lymphatic massage the lymphatics can tend to back up here while doing lymphatic drains and working with the ileocecal valve to help it to relax which in-turn allows it to drain so it's able to function more efficiently.

** *I wrote in chapter twelve an explanation of a self-help technique to help relax your ileocecal valve to drain better.*

* Migrating motor complex (motility issue
* HPA-Axis (motility issue)
* Weak Vagal nerve (motility issue)
* Hypthyroid (motility issue)
* Hormone imbalance (motility issue)
* RO units
* Too many probiotics after fast
* Cavitation
* Reflux meds
* Birth control
* Antibiotics

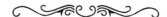

SIBO…Killers

Rotation is a must…

#3		Prokinetics
VIVI		
Cats-a-tonic	*Clove	*BIND
Ec (for E. coli)	*Oregano	*Ginger
The Bomb is WO	*GSE	*Triphala
AO (inflammation)	*Berberine	*Fennel
Ga, Gb, #1, NeruoSyn (motility)	*Neem	
P, Ps, D, L, Lb, (for enzyme deficiency)		

**For more detailed information I have a video about SIBO to watch on my website.

SIBO...Diet

No Fiber, No Sugar, No carb, No fruit and No Vegetables...so what's left
Meat and Fat (The Carnivore Diet)
What about low Fodmap foods

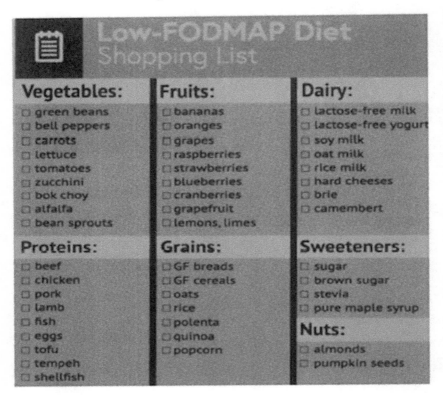

CHAPTER TWELVE

About My Treatments And "My Inspired" Nerve and Tissue Release Technique

In this chapter I am giving you some major self-help techniques without (hopefully) being too overwhelming, you will also find, the instructions for the release of the ileocecal valve that I mentioned before, I also wanted to share with you about an area on top of your feet, for I have found this area to be quite tender and can be extremely painful on those who are suffering acutely from illnesses of any kind which includes headaches, migraines, injuries, energy blocks, sleep issues, and the list goes on. *This is the one and only area on the body that just seems to tackle any and all issues, especially for those of you who suffer from headaches and trouble sleeping.*

My focus as an ND, LMT, CBCP (Naturopathic Doctor, Licensed Massage Therapist & Certified Body Code Practitioner) and Reiki Master is on Migraines, General Body Pain, Back Pain, Sciatica, Autoimmune, Acid Reflux, Sluggish Digestion, Lyme and West Nile Disease, acupressure, muscle balancing, reflexology, polarity balancing, oriental meridians, using food-grade essential oils, essential oil treatments, including rain-drop essential oil therapy, I also do a nerve releasing technique (Nerve Tissue Release Technique), which has been my own discovery through inspiration, that through my experiences may help to balance muscles (which strengthens them), help to relax nerves, and that, in turn, may help alleviate aches and pains as well as the issues listed above including relieving foot pain, that I find so many people suffer from. The Nerve Tissue Release

Technique may also be helpful in releasing illnesses such as viruses and bacterial issues due to better circulation which in-turn allows the nerves to do their job. I find through my own personal experience that it allows my nerves not only to drain, and for the tight muscles to not only relax immediately but also allows the lymphatics to drain more efficiently.

> *The first treatment is generally an hour and a half to three hours, depending on how chronic one's condition is and also depending on if I do a Body Code Session.*

I have discovered through doing bodywork I am empathic therefore I have developed and learned to trust my intuitive gifts and inspirations as well as muscle testing to help guide me through the healing processes coupled with healthy nutrition, herbal remedies, food-grade essential oils along with Systemic Formulas products that are professional-grade supplements that work on a cellular level, and they also have developed their own essential oil combinations. I also will do muscle testing to see what the body needs in priority as far as bodywork goes, essential oils, supplements and also what foods the body may have sensitivities to.

> *Every treatment plan is designed for each individual's needs.*

There are acupressure points that El used when she did the treatments for autoimmune that I found to be very useful towards winning the battle of Lyme and West Nile disease. This treatment also alleviated the fibromyalgia pain I had that seems to accompany Lyme and West Nile, as well as strengthening and stabilizing my energy levels, which helped to kick my body into a healing mode. After experiencing the acupressure treatments that my friend El gave me, I began using those same treatments on my clients who suffered from Lyme or West Nile and who also experienced the same results as I did.

I had started noticing that many people who suffer from Lyme and West Nile experience lymphatic drainage issues, as well as the organ's drain lobes, becoming sluggish which causes even more discomfort. That is when I began to devise over time a treatment plan that helps to retrain the body's memory and ability to regain function in the lymphatic and digestions systems. I will add here for the reader's awareness about what I have seen and how I worked with people who had congestive heart failure, I realized that it was always their left legs that were swollen due to fluid retention. So after releasing and coaxing the lymphatic drains to open a little every day, I began seeing positive results in their healing process and the fluid retention diminishing till finally, their leg was back to a normal state. *I must state here that the reason for not overdoing the draining of lymphatics is that the body can only handle just so much detoxing before causing harm to the liver.* Which I have actually witnessed by someone using an automatic lymph drain pump they had ordered online. This particular individual told me that after he put the pump around his ankle, he unintentionally dropped off to sleep for two hours. He then proceeded to tell me what happened to his liver and to show me what it looked like after he woke up, which to me it resembled a big water balloon for it had swollen clear out from under his rib cage. In which case, I never saw him again. I have also seen people turn a deep orange-yellow color by someone who forced the lymph to drain too much to fast. To put it gently, they also did not heal from their issues. This is why it is so important to know that the therapist who you are allowing to drain the lymph system for you has had actual hands-on training for lymphatic massage. After working with clients for some time who have been suffering from Lyme or West Nile I realized, depending on how chronic their illness was, I would need to do follow up treatments every other day for a week or two *(depending on how their energy was holding)* then the following week I do a treatment every two days and then the next week every three days till the client only needs a treatment once or twice a month, again depending on each individual needs. In very severe cases I may do a treatment once or even twice a day to coax the energy to stabilize and to start holding on its own. My goal in this treatment is to stabilize the energy and to retrain the memory of the body's digestive and lymphatic drainage systems. As research shows, if things are backed up, that's when a decline in a person's health takes place.

Along with treatments, depending on once again how chronic a person may be, the more rest you can get *(this means refrain from any exercising and/or overdue stress)* the better your energy will stabilize and you will heal more sufficiently, the reason I say this is due to my own experience with Lyme and West Nile the more rest I could get the better I would feel. As I have noticed when people expend their energy on resting instead of using their energy on anything else during treatments, they too, heal and regain their energy and strength at a faster and more stable rate.

As for my diet I stay on a strict healthy diet of dark greens and fresh fruit *(staying away from iceberg lettuce)* and I do a bit of juicing with fresh vegetables *(if I use a fruit in my green juice I will only use a small amount as not to have too much sugar on board)*. I do stay away from chicken due to causing allergic reactions such as muscle pain and muscle stiffness. I had even started noticing that when I would work on someone right after lunch who had eaten chicken, it would cause my muscles to tighten and pain to set in which was so bad at times I would have to stop what I was doing to go take some pain meds to be able to continue working! Due to having no pain at all before working on someone who had eaten chicken for lunch, I started putting two an two together by asking them what they had for lunch and 100% of the time they said chicken! I know it sounds crazy, which goes to say everything is energy and gives off energy. That goes for even certain stores or isles in the grocery store! So be aware! For example, here's an account of a client who's friends had recommended that he come to see me. Who was experiencing paralysis, numbing, and tingling sensations on his right side. This particular person had been diagnosed by a neurologist who informed him that he had an extremely rare nerve disease that had a name to it, which I believe used every letter in the alphabet!

This particular person, who happens to be a rancher, appeared to me to be a very healthy individual. His back from my point of view was showing no signs of any disabilities at all. So from there, I started muscle testing his meridian's on his right side to see where the energy blocks were located. Also, I noticed that he had a very deep pocket in his overalls, so I asked him if he was carrying any keys in his pocket his response was a "yes" as he proceeded cleaning out his pocket on his right side he began pulling out tools and of course his chewing tobacco. After he cleaned out his pocket, I then proceeded to muscle test his meridians on the right side once again, which proved that he was much stronger just from clearing out all the metal and tobacco, out of his pocket! That proved to me these items were the root cause of his issues, with overtime, was debilitating to his nervous system. From there, I began doing energy work to create balance in those particular meridians by releasing the blocks I felt in his energy field on his right side. I also did some spinal work by releasing the facet joints on his spinous processes, which in turn helps to release the pressure off the nerves. Just from that one treatment, he started feeling tingling in his right hand, and fingertips which he was not doing before, and the numbness and his leg and foot he was experiencing started diminishing.

I saw this gentleman four more times, the last time I saw him, he was running down the steps as he was leaving and jogging to his truck with a big smile on his face I haven't seen him since. End of story.

My point for sharing these accounts with you is to caution you about what you're carrying on your person or wearing around your wrist and even your fingers, toes, ears*(all the earrings I see people put in the ears all the outer edge is the brain, head, and up the spine and to the shoulder), and navel(which happens to right in the center of the conception vessel meridian!)* Plus, once again I wanted to bring this issue to your attention to help you understand how different energies and frequencies can help you or negatively affect your health. When I see all the earrings in a person's ears, I proceed to ask how their back, neck, and shoulders feel *the answer as you probably guessed...("Not so good.")* For I have had clients who I had been working on, to help them with their low energy and health issues, that after seeing these particular clients for some time, they expressed to me that their energy had started to "go south" on them. When these particular clients would walk into the office, I happen to notice they were wearing a new tool on their wrist that measures their body functions. So I would muscle test it for them to see how it was affecting them energetically. So far, hundred percent of the time, I find these specific devices dramatically diminishes a person's energy level. And as far as acupressure points and meridians *(the energy pathways through the body)* watches and any type of electronic device that a person wears around their wrist lays right on top of a significant acupressure point which has to do with circulation and reproductive organs that also happens to be a triple heater meridian acupressure/acupuncture point.

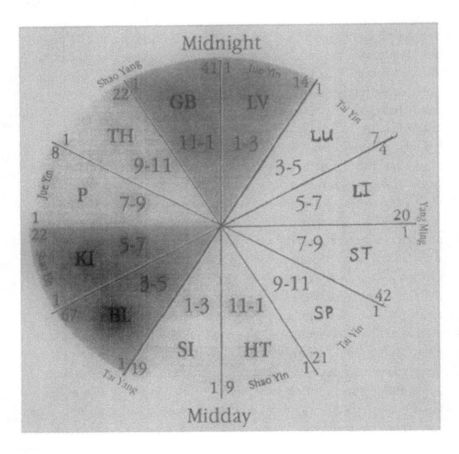

Illustration 1: The chart above shows the Horary Clock which is a Chinese Acupuncture "Meridian Clock" or "Organ Clock". Below are the descriptions of each time phase for each organ.

By checking a meridian chart out, you will see what I am referring to. You can also find much research concerning these issues online. As well as talking to your alternative care doctors about checking to see how these devices may be affecting you, such as your chiropractor and other alternative care specialists who know how to muscle test, I know they would be more than happy to help you with this matter.

Although, in my experience, while such energetic healing devices such as magnets (including different makes) may be okay for the general public, then once again on the flip side of the coin they may not be so "good" for those of us who are highly sensitive or very ill. So when people ask me is this device "good" for me, my reply is, "let's check it out."

This next account is of an elderly lady who came to see me who acquired a drop foot after minor surgery. She informed me a nerve had gotten bruised during the operation and had absolutely no ability to move it even a hair, which required her to use a hook to pull her specialty made boot on. Through numerous treatments over a period of a couple of years, she was once again able to wear a regular flatheeled shoe, which resulted in fewer visits to see me. She hasn't had to come into to see me for nearly a year now due to feeling great. In one of her next to last visits when she came to see me, I had been in the last stages of finishing up the Body Code certification class. When she came in to see me, her complaint was that her foot and leg were aching and she was having a bit of trouble picking the foot up all the way when she took a step. So as I said a little prayer, asking for guidance on what to do for her. I was prompted to give her a symbol of mine *(that I had started drawing a day after I had a particular dream)* to put in her shoe when she went to take a step to our amazement she was able to lift that foot up! And to this day she is still able to lift that foot as she walks! To my way of thinking, the symbol apparently helped her electrical system. From there, I finished up her Body Code treatment and sent her on her way, watching her walk, and thanking the Lord for answering my prayer, as she was leaving.

Okay, more about my symbol that I started drawing the day after I had this particular dream I had years previously while I still had my corn dog shop and this was when I was at the forefront of losing it. I was prompted to draw this particular symbol whenever I felt I could not endure another day of experiencing the feelings of impending doom, that was due to losing what I had worked so hard for as well as experiencing the loss of hope and dreams I had of franchising my shop. So after I started building a clientele in Wyoming, I was prompted to use my symbol to help others by giving it to them to wear on their person or to even charge their water, food, or supplements with. Which I must share with you, that I also put it into the labels of my face cream "Facial Magic" to help enhance its energy moreover, this is the reason I'm sure why it gives a person "nice mellow feel" as they're applying it to their skin.

I have realized through muscle testing plus doing Body Code treatments for myself that Lyme disease made me very sensitive to foods and smells. While with West Nile I've noticed it has caused extreme sensitives to, too many carbohydrates eaten in a day, which in turn I've been noticing more and more that they cause intense brain fog and I've also been noticing the brain fog begins when I've only eaten approximately fifty-five carbs in a day! I've started noticing if I eat over a hundred, then my brain really starts to rebel!

Taking these next products I'm about to mention, and cutting way back on my carb intake a day has really helped and continues to help rid my brain of the rest of the fog I have been suffering with for way to long. The Lyme and West Nile have actually triggered me to have reduced energy as well as emotionally sensitive than normal, in which case I've noticed I've had very little resistance to stress you might say in-which case forces me to need to relax as well as sleep more often than before I started taking the Systemic Formulas products. This too, is why I'm so very grateful that Systemic Formulas has come out with the Ketabo Shake and Extracellular Ketones. Along with these products I also make sure I continue taking the Synulin, two capsules, three times a day along with DSIR Intergen: Which has been Formulated to support the Stomach-Duodenal-Thyroid triad which is foundational to health in Traditional Chinese Medicine. In the last year and half since I've started taking Systemic Formulas' products and started to watch my carb intake I no longer even consider taking naps, unless I've had a few major busy days back to back. And I thought I would never be able to say this!!!

Ketabo Shake: The Ketabo-Shake provides highest-quality, core-level, broad-range, ingredientexpansive nutrition for people who want to boost their dietary diversity while adhering meticulously to the macro-nutrients that support ketogenesis—the production of ketones (acetoacetate, betahydroxybutyrate, and acetone) from fatty acids that serve the body for abundant brain energy and cellular fat-burning for mitochondrial-produced energy.

Extracellular Ketones: BHB, Exogenous ketones are powerful regulators of cellular longevity and directly support both brain and muscle metabolic activities. This Extracellular Ketones formula provides stabile ketones, easily processed in the body into free â-hydroxybutyrate (âOHB) and the free elemental calcium, magnesium, and sodium salts so beneficial to cellular function. For people adapting to, and maintaining, a ketogenic energy supply, supplementing with Extracellular Ketones provides fuel for cellular energy and supports fat-burning cellular metabolic activities.

Since I've begun to watch my carbs more closely, I'm finally able to drop weight easier, which I have been able to do after I started taking the products I mentioned above along with the WO (China Healing Oil) when I would begin to feel like I needed something to eat around three o'clock in the afternoon (which happens to be the small intestine time on the Horary clock) I've started taking five drops of the WO oil which has even helped to curb my discomfort of carb cravings at this time.

The Horary clock is a Chinese Acupuncture "Meridian Clock" or "Organ Clock." There are twelve main meridians, that qi flows through in a twenty-four hour period. You will find a chart and explanations on the times that each meridian comes into play in the following pages. But, first I want to share more information with you about the WO oil, which to my surprise I found it so very amazing in the fight against pain, by releasing those stubborn acupressure points as well as helping my lymphatics drain more efficiently. Besides applying just a drop to my ears and massaging it to the front, and back of the ear (at the center back of the ear where it connects to the head is a point that correlates to the Vegas nerve). And applying it especially to the ear lobes which correlates to the whole head and brain. I apply a bit to my eyebrows as well. I also apply a drop around the naval area, low abdominal *(where a lot of people complain about where fat deposits tend to hang on to a bit too much)*, thyroid, sternum and under the collarbone *(clavicle)*, breast areas as well on the sides of the breast where the bra seams are. I also apply it to the lateral sides of my legs between the hip and knee where you can find three to four major tender points which I make sure I apply a drop to each one of them. This area also correlates with the large intestine and is where a lot of lymph nodes congregate. I know you must be thinking it's going to take a whole bottle a day to apply to all the areas I mentioned, although to my amazement a drop goes a long way! For example, the drops I apply to the three acupressure points I mentioned, to the sides of my legs, I then proceed to massage the excess oil into the rest of the side of my leg. And as for the ears, I divide a drop between them by putting a drop on a finger then tapping that drop with a finger from the other hand, then apply. I must confess that I did go through a whole bottle the first week *(for I did use quite a few drops on my left leg)* which not only helped me to feel better overall, I also noticed an increase in my energy and stamina likewise. I've experienced a lot of pain in my left leg for about twenty years due to getting it bumped pretty hard in a couple of wrecks *(this was due to someone who was not paying attention)*, and since I started using the WO oil on my leg the pain area has dramatically diminished in that first week of applying the WO oil! A couple of my friends who are body-workers had also worked a lot on my left leg which did keep me from excruciating pain and from walking with a cane...which I was envisioning of doing before I meant WO oil. I always felt if I could work on myself every day, I would have no pain, no sluggish lymphatic issues or no low energy and plus back to my original weight, which was my size five western jeans much sooner!! Why is that? You may be asking..."the reason is, so I wouldn't be such a burden on my dear friends causing them to run in the other direction when they see me coming!"

If you look at a meridian chart, you will see that part of the gall-bladder and stomach meridians are on the sides of your legs. There is a gallbladder point on the side of the legs close to the center between your hip and knee that has to do with migraines, and I feel it also has to do with overall general pain and illness. I find this point, along with other points in this area between the hip and knee to be excruciatingly painful on people *(as well as myself)* who are suffering or who has been afflicted by any type of illness, accidents, and/or headaches in their lives.

When I do treatments for anyone I always look out for these particular points, if they happen to be tender at all, I make sure I release them which in my own personal experience helps the person to feel better and may help aid in better circulation and healing. Trust me when I say I know just how painful these areas are and how important it is to have these points released in which I found that by doing my nerve release technique then applying the WO oil I've personally have had the best results than any other type of treatments such as acupressure, and yes, this even includes acupuncture, massage, fascia release, and muscle balancing are among some of the numerous treatments I've had to try to release the pain, and tightness from these particular areas and points.

So trust me when I say that the WO oil is a miracle all on its own! And yes, I have found "first hand" to be in no comparison... and I must say here too that "I have found first hand...it's even far better to combat pain with than a $150.00 bottle of CBD oil!"

In very severe cases I may do a treatment at least once or even twice a day to coax the energy to start holding on its own more than just a few hours. My goal in this treatment is to stabilize the energy and to retrain the memory of the body's digestive and lymphatic drainage systems. As research shows, if things are backed up, that's when a decline in a person's health takes place.

*5 am to 7 am: This is the time of the Large Intestine making it a perfect time to have a bowel movement and remove toxins from the day before. Large intestine, may be cause, to nose bleed, colds, stuffed nose, tooth ache, sore throat, pain in shoulder or arms, swollen belly, diarrhea, dysentery. By massaging your scalp especially tapping between the eye brows helps to clear blocked energy from the mind. At this time, you could also experience emotions of defensiveness, feelings of being stuck or stubbornness could be trapped in the large intestine.

*7–9am: The time of the Stomach…is important to eat the biggest meal of the day here to optimize digestion and absorption. Warm meals that are high in nutrition are best in the morning. May involve issues such as, swollen abdomen, stomach pain, heart burn, vomiting, hunger pains, nose bleed, teeth, chest, menstrual problems, eye and mouth problems, tonsillitis, chest pains, genital pains. Emotions that are likely to be stirred at this time include disgust or despair which also can be trapped which in-turn may may be responsible for indigestion as well as other digestion issues.

*9–11am: This is the time of the Pancreas and Spleen, where enzymes are released to help digest food and release energy for the day ahead. They also involve immune system, edema, genital, connective tissue. Burping, swollen abdomen, stomach pain, heart burn, vomiting, mouth problems, pain in the root of the tongue. This is the ideal time to exercise and work. Do your most taxing tasks of the day at this time. Emotions such as low self-esteem may be felt at this time as well as trapped in these organs.

*11am–1pm: Is the time of the Heart which will work to pump nutrients around the body to help provide you with energy and nutrition. May be the cause of heart problems, insomnia, sweating at night, dry throat, thirst, pain in arms, warm and sweaty palms. Mental, heart, tongue, throat, sleep, emotions This is also a good time to eat lunch and it is recommend to have a light, cooked meal. Having a one hour nap or a cup of tea is also recommended during this time. You may experience feelings of extreme joy or sadness at this time.

*1–3pm: The Small Intestine time and is when food eaten earlier will complete its digestion and assimilation. This is also a good time to go about daily tasks or exercise. Can involve deafness, yellow eyes, sore throat, swollen cheeks, swollen and pain in lower abdomen, frequent urination, often shoulder and arm pains. Ears, throat, small intestine, heart. This is also the time when, vulnerable thoughts or feelings of abandonment may subconsciously arise at this time as well as harbor these emotions.

*3–5pm: The Bladder time when metabolic wastes move into the kidney's filtration system. This is the perfect time to study or complete brain-challenging work. Incontinence, mental problems, malaria, pain in eyes, tearing when windy, nose bleeds, headache, pain in neck and lower back pain. Nose, eyes, urogenital, cramps, pain in shoulder blades and low back. Another cup of tea is advised as is drinking a lot of water to help aid detoxification processes. Feelings of being irritated or timid can also occur at this time.

*5–7pm: The Kidneys time are when the blood is filtered and the kidneys work to maintain proper chemical balance. Incontinence, impotence, menstrual problems, paralyses, edema, sweat, bones, cartilage, nails, hair, ears, asthma, nose bleed, dry tongue sore throat, edema, pain in low back and inside of thighs, warm sweaty feet. This is the perfect time to activate your circulation either by walking or stretching. Subconscious thoughts of fear or terror can also be held in the kidneys.

*7–9pm: Pericardium is responsible for circulation, brain and reproductive organs. This is when nutrients are carried to the capillaries and to each cell. Heart problems, chest cramps, swollen face, swollen armpits, cramp in arms, warm sweaty hands, heart, stomach, motion sickness, mental. This is the perfect time to read. Avoid doing mental activities at this time. A difficulty in expressing emotions may also be felt however, this is the perfect time to have sex or conceive.

*9–11pm: The Triple Heater or endocrine system where the body's homeostasis is adjusted and enzymes are replenished. Swollen abdomen, edema, incontinence, tinnitus, face pain, sore throat, ears, eye problems, pains in the side of chest, midriff, back, constipation, thighs or legs. It is recommended to sleep at this time so the body can conserve energy for the following day. Feelings of paranoia or confusion may also be felt.

*11pm–1am: This is the time of the Gall Bladder and in order to wake feeling energized the body should be at rest. Headache, jaw problems, vision, bitter taste in mouth, pain in shoulder blades, armpits, down the side of the body and lower back, eyes, hips, seat. In Chinese medicine, this period of time is when yin energy fades and yang energy begins to grow. Yang energy helps you to keep active during the day and is stored when you are asleep. Trapped emotions of resentment may appear in the gall bladder.

*1–3am: The time of the Liver is time when the body should be asleep. During this time, toxins are released from the body and fresh new blood is made. Pain in lower abdomen headache, hernia, dry throat, hiccups, incontinence, mental problems. Liver, urogenital, eyes, muscles, spleen sinew. If you find yourself waking during this time, you could have too much yang energy or problems with your liver or detoxification pathways. If you wake up at this time your liver is overwhelmed by the detoxing process. Such as alcohol, chemicals, drugs, poor diet all need detox by liver. This is when we do our deep sleeping and dreaming. The liver can also hold on to trapped emotions of frustration and anger.

*3–5am: The time of the Lungs and again, this is the time where the body should be asleep. If woken at this time, nerve soothing exercises are recommended such as breathing exercises. Cough, asthma, sore throat, pressure in chest, pain in shoulders, neck and arms. Lungs, breathing, skin, throat, neck, The body should be kept warm at this time too to help the lungs replenish the body with oxygen. The lungs are also associated with feelings of grief and sadness and can also hold on to these emotions.

I cut out all processed foods including going out to eat, and any premixed spices (unless the ingredients are all herbs) including all boxed or packaged mixes. I also cut out chicken (I've noticed it can cause undue pain I did research on allergies to chicken which I found can cause stomach issues and pain) As far as eggs go…the trend to eating right is to go for the organic eggs, I do generally buy the range free eggs. I found when I eat the some "organic" eggs they upset my digestion and feelings of nausea set in. I also stay away from potatoes, although I do eat baked sweet potatoes. I find the longer I am on whole foods which also includes fish, pork, beef, along with a green salad (that includes spinach, kale, and chard for its base) I have noticed too when I am very busy in my shop and go for a couple of days without my greens my energy starts to diminish.

I have come to the realization after finally figuring it out which has taken a few years on how to keep going…just how important stabilizing your energy is and that it's "the main key" to my surviving Lyme and west Nile.

Below is a text message from a very dear friend who came to stay with me for a few days, due to not feeling well for a couple of years caused from some digestive issues. She expresses her challenges about how difficult it is to eat better for your health. She also mentioned she used her microwave everyday. Which is one thing I stay away from at all cost! For it is one of the many things I find that the food from the microwave causes me immense heartburn, Which I have noticed through the years that it seems to affect others in the same way. So you might want to seriously consider what you eat and how you prepare your food before ingesting it if you are not feeling well and/or stomach and digestive issues.

The reason for sharing this with you is that when someone comes in to see me with complaints of stomach upset of any kind, the two things I ask first is, "do you drink ice cold water or ice cold drinks of any kind and the second question is, do you use a micro-wave to cook your food?"

Janee: Hello my friend. Just thinking of you today. Are you in Idaho or Wyoming working? I've been taking my supplements faithfully. Not eating perfect though. Argh!! It's so hard! I must say I felt so much better and more like myself than I have for some time now! Thank you for your help!"

Me: "Oh my. I was going to check in on u today!! I am in Idaho. Want to come up!?

How are u feeling?

Heads up The unhealthy foods will only plug you up more, and will not allow your body to heal. For your encouragement,

I didn't eat, not even a taste of chocolate for two years! Or anything I wasn't supposed to. That the doctor

In Vegas told me I should not eat after testing my allergies.

I was taught that It takes seven months to make all new blood cells and years for a whole new body. It just takes a long time and endurance on eating a healthy diet, to heal.

I know how hard it is to eat right how much time it takes to fix. We are in a battle against corrupt

nutrition that destroys valuable quality of life.

It's Not what most of us were taught growing up…"take a pill you'll be fine. It doesn't matter what you eat…or drink…"

I am very grateful I am able to be of help!

I must say, I hear a lot of these types of stories in my office. Therefore, so that you know, you are not alone with these eating and health challenges, and this is one of the many reasons I am here is to help and encourage you on your journey to a healthier you.

People will ask me, how do I know where the sore spots are. All I can say is, besides following my instincts I have had the same pains in the same places and also in my practice I find most everyone has the same pains who are not feeling well. And I too am still battling somewhat with the scarring of Lyme and west Nile.

By integrating the different modalities, together we can work towards helping you achieve your goals.

I have studied many different modalities, some of which includes Muscle Balancing and other energy work techniques, for the last fifteen years.

I also have worked in an alternative care clinic for close to seven years prior to building my own practice.

I have put together techniques that includes a nerve release technique that may help pain in general including foot pain, leg pain, migraines, back pain, sciatica, and muscle pain.

Interested in classes for my
Nerve Tissue Release Technique? You will find
contact information at the end of this book

I must share with you one of the most disturbing questions people ask me which is "Where and what type of therapist or doctor do I need to find that does what you do?"

My response is, "I experience the best results when I have lymphatic work done, acupressure for any type autoimmune diseases, and polarity balancing to re-balance the individual organs and, my elements (fire, water, earth, mental, and wood), reflexology, and cranial sacral."

And now that I have the fortitude of having my Nerve Tissue Release Technique done for me, and a supplement regimen which I use the Body Code to figure out what supplementation I need, plus I also test for the quantity I need each day, and how many bottles my body requires of each supplement, tincture or of a particular herb. These are the modalities that have helped to heal my body from Lyme and West Nile over and above any other treatments or therapy's.

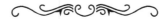

By now you are most likely thinking "who does all of that in one session?" *I do if needed.* And by muscle testing or using The Body

Code I test to see what the body needs in priority. The reason I know this is due from having had El in my life, and other therapist that I've meant through my classes, and being taught by one of the very best instructors out there.

And so you know, there are other bodyworkers out there that do combine these particular modalities together during a session you just have to do some searching and asking questions.

I have been asked this question almost everyday while at work, by the people who would come for treatment with all different types of issues from leg pains, sciatica, migraines, to all forms of cancer, and so on, these people would come from all parts of the country. The people whom I had the honor of doing treatments for, and who often stayed for a day or even weeks, as they would come in every day for treatments, they would ask me if I was going to do the bodywork treatments for them. So while I was giving them a treatment they would whisper to me that they didn't know what treatments were doing the most good for them, then they proceeded to say to me "all I know is, when you don't work on me I don't feel as well, with just having the standard treatments offered to me." And as for the "victims of cancer," I would do a Polarity treatment "for all forms of Cancer." Whenever I would do this type of treatment, these individuals made certain to let me know they felt much better the following day than they have been feeling for some time and they always asked if I would do more treatments for them.

As every person understands, when you have rave reviews for your work, then you know to keep doing what you're doing. Encouragement, support, and inspiration from others gives us the confidence to continue to learn, and develop our talents, skills, and abilities, so we feel more confident to continue on with our missions, objectives, and goals in life.

Whenever I am asked this question, my heart goes out to those people, and this is one of many reasons for building my own clientele, for it gives me the ability to take as long as necessary to do a treatment for a client, and to do as many sessions as they require.

So what I was hearing from all this information, is that there needs to be more "bodyworkers" available to do these types of therapies such as I have had the fortune to learn and to blend the different modalities during a treatment.

I also hear a lot of these same stories from my clients when they share their experiences of trying to get their issues resolved or at least headed in a better direction than they had been going. As I've mentioned before I do know how it feels to be sent out the door after an evaluation and treatment with realization setting in that my ongoing issue of not feeling well is not any closer to being resolved, and at the same time I don't feel any better when I left than I did before I walked in.

My goal is to help people become pain free *(in-which I also tune into my intuitive gifts)* therefore I rarely do massages, for they may only last two or three days if that, then the pain returns. I say this from my own personal experiences.

I also use the Body Code to help identify and locate where the basis of the issue lies and also may help to release those unwanted emotional burdens that may be causing you not only emotional disturbances but also may be causing physical pain as well.

The Body Code is where we identify and correct imbalances that can cause emotional and physical problems for people and also for animals as well. The body has powerful abilities to heal if conditions are right and the Body Code makes it simple to find those underlying imbalances easily and quickly. The Body Code also enables me to do distant healing *(through proxy)* for people and animals.

I have debated about sharing the following experiences with you due to alienating some of you who have difficulty to fully understand extra sensitive people's different gifts and the unseen energies we may experience in our lives. Due to these issues, it causes us to keep those gifts to ourselves so as not to cause undue emotional stress for ourselves or to those who require scientific explanations for…the unexplainable experiences people have, and for those who choose not to understand that there are energies in this awesome world of ours which even modern science is not able to tune into or explain. And this is why I felt impressed upon to share some of my "let's just say sci-fi" experiences so as not to eliminate those of us who are "extra sensitive" and that do have an understanding of unexplainable gifts, and experiences. With that said, next is a couple of Body Code treatments I want to share with you in-which these treatments even surprised me!

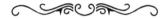

I have found after some time of doing Body Code treatments for people I've discovered I have become more aware of my gifts such as learning that I am sensitive in being able to feel if a client's deceased relative is following them to my office. During the Body Code session, I have found that their relatives happen to be in need of a Body Code treatment as well! Which has happened a few times during someone's Body Code session. For instance, one client, in particular, comes to mind who had a disembodied spirit (ghost) you might say, follow her into the office, and during the client's Body Code session, this disembodied spirit interrupted me during the session. The timing was surprising to me when this spirit decided to interrupt me! For it was right on cue! After I found out during the Body Code session that my client had trapped emotions due to a disembodied spirit *(ghost)* following her, the next question I asked, I found the spirit to be a female cousin of hers. Right then I felt it was time to pause the session with my client to do a Body Code session for her "spirit" cousin. First off, I found during the Body Code session the spirit had trapped emotions of unworthiness and confusion. Then next, I found she had a Sabature that had not only had suffered emotional harm I also discovered she suffered physical harm as well due to an energy weapon that happened to be a bullet! Then I asked my client to confirm if what I was picking on, happened to be correct. With a nod of her head, my client proceeded to share with me through tears of hidden emotions, of how her cousin's boyfriend had shot and killed her during one of their many arguments! After I finished her treatment, she was then able to go to the Light, creating a very peaceful, beautiful aura in the room as she was leaving.

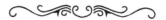

In another session that stands out is about a friend of mine who also comes to see me as a client. During one of her visits to my office, she happened to be accompanied by a grandmother, from the other side who had experienced a lot of pain in her feet while alive. This grandmother wanted to know why her feet bothered her so much. How I discovered her feet issue during her life was through the Body Code session I did for her. Come to find out she had a problem with a particular vein in the lower extremities of her legs causing swelling and poor circulation in her feet and ankles. I asked my friend if her grandmother had suffered from a lot of pain in her feet during her life. My friend informed me her grandmother had suffered a lot during her life due to swelling and inflammation in her lower extremities which caused her a lot of pain in her feet, and no one could figure out why her feet bothered her so much. She too left leaving a "light soft" aura feeling in the room.

—————————For everything is Energy!—————————

To give you an idea of what a body code treatment involves. I will share with you one of many body code treatments I have done for myself. I happened to listen to a class in-which I will call "business energies," so I thought I would give myself a body code treatment for business energies.

Here goes: Using the Body Code techniques I found my business energies frequency was functioning at only one percent.

So after I tested for why my business energies I found they were almost non-functional, I found that I had an inherited 63% generational old, trapped emotion of stubbornness that I inherited from my dad's, mom's side who's heritage is of English and Irish origin. What happened next was as soon as I found the lineage of where this trapped emotion came from, to my amazement, I instantly felt a sensation, of a stabbing, numbing, tingling pain and tightness on my left shoulder halfway between the tip of my shoulder and edge of neck along the upper trap muscle. Then I felt that same sensation continue up my neck following the path of the upper trap muscle which involves colon and eyes. Amazing! So after clearing the stubbornness trapped emotion I then asked what percentage my business energies were functioning. I found they escalated up to functioning at eighty-seven percent. As I proceeded with my treatment I found I had an inherited an anger trapped emotion which I found through testing was located in my liver and also the liver meridian in my left leg in-which I found came from the same sixty-three generational *(a generation is twenty years)* grandmother. As I was releasing this sixty-three generational trapped emotion of an anger issue, oddly enough, just in the area above the knee half way up on the inside of my left leg is where I have always experienced a lot of pain and discomfort in that section of my liver meridian!

This all makes since due to having horrible leg aches in my childhood as young as I can remember till I was about five years old. Then that's about the time where I found I could just ignore the pain, after all it's the thing you have to do being a little farm girl. A lot of you who suffer with pain I'm sure you can relate.

Fortunately after releasing the trapped emotion of anger from my liver and liver meridian my business energies were functioning at a hundred percent! I did notice my leg pain started diminishing soon after I finished the treatment and to my amazement my leg continued to feel better throughout the day. With these body code treatments they can take a few days to totally process which includes not only physical processing but emotional as well.

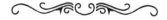

*I am petitioning all Body-Workers who have these skills, and who are **"Passionately Dedicated"** in helping and learning **"my format"** to help battle against Lyme & West Nile, to email me with your business contact information. I will add you to a business directory on my website for the people who are looking for a Therapist in their area*

that uses the modalities listed above. Lets Work as a Team to Help Fight the battle of pain and suffering from Lyme and West Nile.

*Disclaimer: No representation contained in these materials is intended as medical advice and should not be used for diagnosis or medical treatments.

CHAPTER THIRTEEN

The Testimonials Including Jesseca Cross, United States Olympian

I met Kathy Gaa after traveling decades through the typical athlete per-formance/injury/recovery/re-injury/aging timeline. I am a 2000 United States Olympian who currently has a career in health, fitness, coaching, and nutrition. I spent many years in pain though I thrived in athletics.

Over time the chronic use of the nervous and muscular systems I have led to constant adhesions and injury in the same old places. As an elite athlete I was given many modalities of treatment and all of them helped in certain points during my career. When I met Kathy I was exposed to the pain free way of treating the human body. Kathy's approach is holistic driven and comes from many years of learning and applying throughout her lifetime. She shared her per-sonal story with me about her sickness and injuries and I connected with her instantly. She has and continues to reach into the depths of my decades of sports and back in the day nutrition fads (I do not use these any longer though the residue of what we ingest physically and emotionally reside with us always).

Kathy has undone some of the things in me that I had not found relief to as well as connecting the sources of pain and disruption. She has aided my digestion, sleep, awareness, and calmness. She is dedicated to finding what is best for each person she meets. She is not a quick fix. What she does not know she will learn to know in order to help anyone be well. Her personality brightens the room and her knowledge is not of the majority...meaning she holds the tickets to modalities that most do not know. The modalities work. She is patient and encouraging. The best characteristic about her is the excitement she shows when her work brings healing to me. She is a gift to the world.

Jesseca Cross
United States Olympian

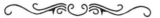

Endorsement: Kathy Gaa, is truly an individual with strong energy and insight. Her knowledge and experience of how the body systems, mind, soul and spirit work in correlation is remarkable! She has helped me in numerous ways to overcome past experiences that were not favorable, and brought forward the positive light of the present thru acupressure, massage and body code. Thank you Kathy—I will always remember what you've done for me in my life!

Erica Loloff

To Whom It may concern:

My name is Kassia Alexander. I am writing to say that I have known and worked with Kathy for almost 8 years. She is an awesome massage therapist and so much more. She would always go the extra mile for our patients often staying late to care for them. She always put the patient first. I really loved working with her and miss her now that she is gone. She is missed by so many of our patients. She helped so many people and I feel that she truly has a healing gift.

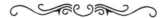

Thank you to my friend Kathy. She knows her stuff. And mine also! Kathy takes time to listen, perform her knowledge and then does what her hands and mind asked her to do. I personally suffer from a situation too real to talk about and I personally feel much better after several treatments. My body is measurably smaller due to her opening pathways for function to return. I walk taller and with more confidence. Listen with your ears and brain when she says words from out of the blue. "Microwave" "Toe ring" are words that make me silent and laughing at our history. Lol.

Kathy is a talented healer. She is a listener. A gentle friend. My body feels refreshed. My mind open to history and the future. She treats me with wisdom, knowledge and kindness. She treats my body with knowledge, pressure and greatest of respect.

I feel personally honored to be a patient of yours.

A huge shout out and great respect to you my friend Kathy!!

Shirlyn

8/20/2019

Kathy,

I would like to thank you for the way I have been feeling lately, no doctor or chiropractor has been able to help me get back on my feet as you have!! Since my Spine Surgery in 2015 my body has not been the same physically…

Now that I am getting older and still having nerve problems associated with my back & neck which affects my breathing, whole body, and outlook on life…My spine surgery left me with limited range of motion in my neck among other parts of my body as we've talked. I went through the specified time in Physical Therapy, and near the last physical check the therapist in charge actually forced my neck to turn as he thought it should go…I pushed his hand away…but forcing my head made my neck feel as if it was on fire. I feel he re-injured my neck. I was in a lot of pain!!! I did not want the pain pills that was offered to me. I could not afford to go through my day on the job drugged up. I needed to be present mentally and physically at my job…I suffered severe headaches…I just wanted to shut the curtains, crawl in my bed and try to relieve my throbbing headache right after work… which wasn't working for my family…at my house, I am in charge of dinner…I lived on "Excedrin Migraine" about 7 years before my surgery and after…I also had problems with extremities. The left side of my face and neck often went numb or had a burning feeling, same for raising my hands above my head numbness or burning…Before my surgery my Surgeon explained what, I'm experiencing now, could happen or it might be worse…The pain could be temporary or permanent but at the time I was in so much pain I was willing to go along…The condition in my face is similar to Bell's Palsy due to the fact that the doctor had to cut several nerves in my neck to get to my spine…Four years later I am still having the numbing & burning problems…My doctor is nowhere to be found…Most doctors I have been seeing nowadays, seem to repeat what they are trained to do. Over & over they suggest "my band—aid" more physical therapy and more pills. I'm not getting anywhere…except back to them. I feel I have done what the doctors have asked me to do long enough!!!! I am hoping to get as close to being back to my normal…before my life is gone…I'm So thankful I was referred to you, I spoke with you on the phone and then met you, I knew you would be able to help me!!! I felt an instant trust with you, I felt the sincerity you have to help people, and for me that is a big thing…I felt bad because I wasn't doing so well when we met, and if you were going to be able to help me…it was going to be a big job for both of us!!! That day you aligned my spine and untangled a bunch of nerves, for the rest of that day, and for the first time in four years I was on my way to being pain free!!!! Yippee!!!! In the weeks that followed I have not had one single headache!!!! I felt and still feel like a kid again!!! I am soooooo grateful for your knowledge, wisdom, and willingness to help me take better care of myself, so that I am able to work through my physical issues and continue doing all the things that a mother needs to do for her family & job!!! Without pain pills!!!! Thank You for caring, seeing, & knowing, how important it is for me to stay engaged in my life!!! I will always be grateful and continue recommending you a million times over, to anyone who needs an AMAZING Holistic Healer!!!

Thank you!!!

D.P

Protocols Includes Supplement Protocols, Lyme Disease, Parasite Protocols and a GI Purge program

The Capsules you take...are they toxic to your system?

So I did some research about Systemic Formulas capsules I found their capsules do not contain SLS (sodium laureth sulfate), Ti02 (titanium oxide), or sorbic acid which have all been banned by Japan.

Question you may want to ask yourself about the capsules you are taking...are they made with these toxic substances?

When taking 125 mcg of Ti02in about 2 mg per day...highly toxic. As well, each veggie cap contains about 1 mg of SLS (a known cancer causing agent). Imagine downing 20 capsules of veggie caps daily and getting 20mg of SLS internally each day!

This is why I work hard to not eat processed foods, and not to use pre-mixed spices that has additives added to them other than the natural herbs and spices. So to mention a few I stay away from like the Plague are such items as dried taco mixes, gravy mixes, soup mixes, mixes to make your own salad dressings, and the list goes on. The reason for this is due to the ages of people who come into my office that are in their mid forties and upwards especially those who are in their mid to late sixties. For as I do treatments for them that involves digestion issues *(which interestingly happens to be their chief complaint when they come to see me)*, I ask them about their eating habits during their lives. By now, from the information I have shared with you thus far, I'm sure you can tell what kind of diet they have been on. Which is most likely…you guessed it…**"The See Food Diet"** which is self-explanatory…Such as…if it exists then I am going to Eat and/ or Drink it…for My Body is Strong and has been made to withstand any Type of Ice Drinks, and Eatable Substances even though it is mostly made with or totally made of Chemicals or Food that is so over processed there is no food value left in it therefore Chemical Nutrition has to be added and Chemical Food Coloring to make it *"yummy looking"* especially to our children so they will want to eat and drink plenty! So as to stay strong and healthy!

I know this all sounds funny and a bit crazy, but just as I have said before, I am sharing with you what I have personally seen and experienced on a personal level in my own life and the stories about peoples ailments I hear about in my office. *I challenge you to do more research on your own about food* additives and colorings *(may cause muscle pain)*, for I am personally more concerned about ingesting these type substances mentioned above than making sure I'm eating all organic whole foods for I have found the non-organic whole grains and vegetables does not give my head a "zing" as does chemicalized based food products do.

Lyme Instructions

Drainers
Always be on at least 1 drainer at all times. Symptoms occur when the body is not draining the die off and debris out of the body.

- SENG by Systemic Formulas
o   2 caps 2 times a day
- ACX by Systemic Formulas
o   2 caps 2 times a day

Killers

** Take an Option for 12 days, take 2 days off and Pick a DIFFERENT Option**

- Cat's a Tonic by Systemic Formulas
o (Dosage and Use: Start with 1 drop twice in 4 oz. water, under tongue. Slowly increase dosage to 30 drops 3 times daily).
- S Spleen by Systemic Formulas
o 2 caps, 2-3 times a day

- ATAK by Systemic Formulas
o Begin with 2 caps per day and work up to 2 caps, 3 times a day
- MELA by Systemic Formulas
o 2 caps 1-3 times a day on an empty stomach

- GOLD by Systemic Formulas
o 2 caps 2 times a day
§ If you get niacin flush take with food or take only 1 capsule at a time
- Gt Thymus by Systemic Formulas
o 2 caps, 2-3 times a day

- Vitamin C / sea salt (8-16 gm. daily of vitamin c and sea salt (equal doses of each), in 3-4 doses throughout day.) *See below for mechanism of action.
o Stimulates the immune system.
o Effective for the Cell-Wall-Deficient phase.

* Salt, Vitamin C Protocol
- Salt enhances the activity of elastase, an enzyme which contributes to white blood cell function and immunity.
- During acute inflammatory responses, elastase is released by white blood cells called neutrophils.
- The released substance generates fibers in surrounding tissues that may facilitate phagocytosis (the break down and destruc-

tion of pathogens) by trapping bacteria and focusing enzyme activity on their elimination.

- Combined with large doses of Vitamin C, the indirect killing ability of elastase is dramatically increased.
- Second, increasing sodium concentration surrounding micro-organisms like Borrelia Burgdorferi leads to bacterial death as sodium ions enter the spirochete form of the bacterium.
- To be precise, "an increased intracellular sodium concentration, combined with a decreased potassium concentration, leads to spirochete death." Specific cause of death is by activity of an antimicrobial peptide in neutrophils known as LL-37.

In the following charts you will find lists for multi-vitamins, minerals, as well as suggested supplements for different issues, healthy glands and organs.

GI Purge Instructions:15 days: Morning & Evening
2 #3Bactrex with or without food
2 #4 FungDX with or without food
2 ENZEE (away from food)

Before Bed: 6-8 BIND

A Clean Sweep Parasite Program

All things in health revolve around balance—too much or too little causes symptoms or alternate epigenetic expressions of genes (activations/deactivations). Over-sterilization of our environment causes immunological complacency. But the other side of that is the over-toxicity of our environment and the great need to detoxify. The worms, bacteria, virus, and fungus come into our lives because of the internal terrain we provide. The more toxic our body-terrain becomes with chemicals and altered foods, the more the candida-fungus, virus, and bacteria come to our rescue to eat the debris. The worms prefer a weak host and humans become susceptible to their residency when excessive pathogens weaken or occupy the immune system's attention.

Helminths can occupy the immune system's attention so it stops attacking the intestines. But why did the immune system errantly attack the intestines in the first place? It was not a lack of helminths--it was an imbalance in the other factors such as disruption of the innate intestinal flora by antibiotics and a junk food diet. We don't need helminths in our intestines, but we do need 85% beneficial flora and 15% potentially pathogenic flora (to keep the immune system vigilant). Nature has set the ecological niches for all life. The range of balance is wide, but more than ever before, humanity is attempting to control Nature and live outside of its established parameters. Systemic Formulas provides an excellent Pathogen Purge Program to help rid fungus, bacterial, mycoplasma, and virus; a Leaky Gut Program to help strengthen the intestinal integrity and restore the beneficial flora;

Following are the formulas used in the Clean Sweep Parasite Program to help the body get rid of unwanted visitors.

These unique formulations utilize ingredients from many remote areas and set a new standard for the natural approach of maintaining a body free of parasitic influences.

VRM-1 (Large)	addresses large intestinal worms such as tapeworms (Cestoda).
VRM-2 (Small)	addresses small, intestinal and blood-based parasites including roundworms (Nematoda) and microfilaria.
VRM-3 (Micro)	addresses micro-organisms in the intestines such as giardia, C-diff, entamoeba histolytica (Protozoa, Amoeba, and some gram positive bacteria).
VRM-4 (Cell)	addresses mobile parasites such as flukes (Trematoda) as well as those that invade the cells.

| WO (China Healing Oil) | this ancient formula was refined and designed to expel parasites in addition to countless other uses. The WO refers to the rare wormseed oil historically known to be a powerful vermifuge. |

INSTRUCTIONS FOR:
A CLEAN SWEEP PARASITE PROGRAM

For Adults, for 10 days, take:

45 Minutes Before Breakfast (Away From Food, Especially Protein)

If food is needed to take the herb capsules, use celery, carrot, sprouts, etc.

3 capsules VRM-2

3 capsules VRM-4

WO oil—pour into a capsule, take orally

Before Bed (Away From Food, Especially Protein)

3 capsules VRM-1

3 capsules VRM-3

WO oil—pour into a capsule, take orally

Then stop taking the VRM formulas for 5 days. Then resume with a second 10-day cycle. Then abstain from taking the formulas for 5 days. Then do a third 10-day cycle.

Note #1. Some people may need to start with lower doses. This program should be comfortable. If not, lower the dosage and gradually increase to full program.

Note #2: Dead parasites are toxic. As can occur with cleansing processes, the toxins can sometimes make a person irritable. If this occurs, practitioners recommend drinking more water and taking 1 capsule of ACX (Vitamin Detox) three times a day.

Some people may need 4, even 5 cycles to become free of parasites.

The VRM formulas also come in liquid tincture for those who have difficulty swallowing capsules.

In the next following pages you will find a lists of supplements and their intended purposes for the body. If you are unsure of what supplements to take at this time in your life and would like help with determining what your body needs, we can schedule a Body Code treatment which can be done by proxy if you are not wanting to make the trip to come see me. Please feel free to contact me. My contact information is listed in the back of this book as well as my website. www.mountainrosewellnesscenter.com

The Body Code Energy Work is where we identify and correct imbalances that can cause emotional and physical problems for people and animals. The Body has powerful abilities to heal if conditions are right and the Body Code makes it simple to find those underlying imbalances easily and quickly. With the Body Code, I am able to do distant energy healing (through proxy) for body and mind for people and animals. For everything is Energy!

The supplements are listed in thirteen categories. Starting with Bio Command, Bio Function, Bio Nutriment, Bio Extract, BIOME, Bio Challenge, KIDZ Play, Bio Basic, CHINESE 5 ELEMENTS, Bio Cell, Bio Tincture, CX EXTRACTS, PROGRAM PACKAGES.

BIO COMMAND—gives the body an authoritative order

#1-ACTIVATOR—Provides nutrients that support hypothalamic functions

#2-BUILDER—Supports tissues' inherent rebuilding function

#3-BACTREX—Kills bacteria and helps the production of white blood cells

#4-FUNGDX—Kills fungus and slows fungal growth

#5-STABILIZER—Supports proper cellular reproduction and stabilizes functions in the body

#6-RESTORE—Nutrients support cellular integrity and restores functions in the body

BIO FUNCTION—an activity or purpose natural to or intended for the body

#12 B-BRAIN—Nourishes the neuronal cellular matrix; supports the brain's normal processes of concentration

#14 C-COLON—Assists in toning the bowel tissue and supports peristalsis. It is a hydragogue, thus assists with lymphatic and bowel purification

#17 D-DIGEST—Fungal Based Enzyme solution that promotes digestion of proteins, carbohydrates, and fats

#18 DS-DIGEST S—This formula utilizes vegetable enzymes to provide support for good digestive health

#19 DB12—DIGESTIVES + B12—Support the stomach's parietal cells that produce intrinsic factor—a glycoprotein essential for the absorption of Vitamin B12

#22 F+—FEMALE PLUS—Provides nutritional support for healthy female biochemistry, hormonal balance and ovarian/uterine health

#24 FPMS—FEMALE HEALTH—Support to help normalize the menstrual cycle associated with excessive bleeding, hot flashes, mood swings and accompanying dysmenorrhea cramps

#31 GA-ADRENAL—Builds and balances the adrenal glands

#32 GB-PITUITARY/PINEAL—Provides nutritional support for all the important brain glands—pituitary, pineal, and thalamus

#39 GF-THYROID—Builds and balances the thyroid gland

#41 GT-THYMUS—Provides the perfect nutrition for the thymus gland, the immune system's master regulator

#44 H-HEART—Provides nutrients for optimal heart health to strengthen the heart muscle

#45 HCV-HEART CARDIOVASCULAR—Provides nutritional tissue support for the arteries, veins, and capillaries. Supports a healthy circulation and blood pathway integrity

#48 HQ-HEART ENERGY—Total support approach to the heart's energy—Creating and maintaining sustained energy, optimal production of ATP, and optimal cardiac function

#50 I-EYES—Supports the brain's optic center (back lobes); supplies nutrients necessary for clear vision

#56 K-KIDNEY—Kidney support formula for integrity of the kidney tissue. K Kidney is also a great addition to a general bladder health protocol.

#58 KS-KIDNEY S—This formula supports normalized kidney function. Kidney support formula for regulating pH, maintaining electrolyte balance, and contributes nutrients used in the self-cleansing processes

#60 L-LIVER—Liver building formula that supports building & maintenance of the liver's intercellular tissues

#62 LS-LIVER S—Supports the liver's function and provides nutrient cofactors consumed in the liver's innate detoxification processes

#61 LB-LIVER GALLBLADDER—Designed for general liver/gallbladder support and cleansing. Helps the body maintain proper portal duct function

#70 M+-MALE ENDOCRINE—Supports the male glandular and endocrine systems

#72 MPC-PROSTATA CORRECTOR—Prostate support formula that provides nutritional factors that support a healthy prostate gland and healthy circulation

#73 MPR-PROSTATA OVATUM—Support for the male and female reproductive glands as well bursa

#74 N-NERVE—General nerve support for the whole nervous system with specific herbalomic nutriments for nerve support for the bundle branch nerves that serve the heart

#75 N3-RELAXA—Designed for individuals who have feelings of anxiety and disorientation and have difficulty resting due to occasional stress; N3 provides nutrients that support the calming neurotransmitter response of GABA

#78 P-PANCREAS—Supports normal pancreatic functions including production of insulin & glucagons and tissue integrity

#79 PS-PANCREAS S—Bolsters and maintains internal pancreatic balance—helps maintain an already healthy blood glucose level

#80 R-LUNG—Complete Nutritional Lung support. This formula was designed to support a healthy respiratory system and maintain normal mucus levels, as well as to support the oxygen-carrying capacity of the lungs

#82 S-SPLEEN—Nutritional support for the spleen. Supports spleen health which can influence the lymphatic and blood systems as well as the immune system

BIO NUTRIMENT—nourishment and sustenance for the body

#100 ABC-ACID/BIF/BULG/COMP—This formula balances beneficial flora in the gastrointestinal tract. Each capsule contains a minimum of 12-billion enterically-coated spore form probiotics

#101 ACP-VITAMIN ACP—"drainage" remedy and mild cellular detox. Specifically effective for collagen tissue and muscle detox

#102 ACX-VITAMIN DTX—High potency, broad-spectrum detoxifier; an excellent drainage formula for use in any cleansing, elimination program, and/or detoxification program, especially for organ detoxification

#108 ALG-ALGAE OMEGA—Serve the body's inflammation-resolution mechanisms. Support the body's efforts to maintain a positive mood, efficient concentration, memory processes, and cell membrane insulin sensitivity

#111 AZV-MULTIVITAMIN AND MIN—An all purpose, multi-vitamin, mineral and herbal formula that provides particular focus for liver nutrition

#114 BFO-BORAGE/FLAX/FISH OIL—Support healthy blood vessels, joints, and aid in maintenance of healthy cholesterol

#115 B16-16 B VITAMINS—supports bodies ability to adapt to the normal daily stresses of life

#120 CAL-CALCIUM PLUS—Calcium malate and calcium citrate—in a matrix of magnesium malate and citrate with Vitamin D3 and K2 with synergists Zinc, Manganese, Strontium and Boron to assist in maximum assimilation

#123 CLR-CHLOROPHYLLIUM—provides photosynthetic pigment for Pancreatic health and mucus membrane balance

#126 CTV-VITAMIN C—The ultimate Vitamin C complex with ECGC for optimal cellular nutrient uptake.

#128 CVOR-CARDIOVASCULAR OIL—Support healthy cholesterol processes including cholesterol sulfate which is involved in cell membrane integrity and cardiovascular health

#129 DV3-VITAMIN D3 + IMMUNE—Clinically effective supplement for establishing activated vitamin D receptors associated with optimal health

#130 EZV-VITAMIN E—A truly natural Vitamin E provided in a pleasant, chewable form that optimizes assimilation. Powerful antioxidant.

#131 FBR-FIBER—A unique, tasty powder blend of insoluble & soluble fibers plus the power of herbs, whole food organic sprouts, and probiotics. Assists with healthy digestion & elimination of toxins

#132 FLX-FLAX SEED OIL—Sustain healthy levels of cholesterol, and is essential in building and strengthening general glandular and hormonal functions. Contains lignans known to prevent cancer and helps with nerve impulses.

#133 JOT-JOINT, DISC, CARTILAGE—Support cartilage integrity, joint health, lubrication and comfort.

#134 LEV-LECITHIN—Ideal for a healthy brain, heart, nerves, liver, joints and cell membranes.

#138 MBC-MICRO-BIOME COLONIZER—High potency, ten species, enteric-coated, spore form, probiotic formula designed to re-colonize the Gastrointestinal Tract microbiome with beneficial, high attachment species. 100 Billion

#140 MIN-MULTI MINERAL PLUS—Broad-spectrum mineral formula that supports maintenance of the body's electrolytic balance

#150 PRO-NUTRO PROTEIN—Provides essential amino acids and peptide chains commonly deficient in today's average diet; it enhances and completes the dietary proteins

#155 PTM-POTASSIUM STABILIZER—A natural, plant source of two forms of potassium (bitartrate and chloride)

#180 REL-CHLORELLA—supports overall body systems during cleansing programs—useful in heavy metal detoxification programs

#184 ROX-SUPER ANTIOXIDANT—Broad "blanket" approach for whole body support, especially for the arteries and cell membranes. Contains resveratrol for telomere support.

#187 TMI-THYROID METABOLISM—This formula nourishes and supports the thyroid metabolic processes via multi-source iodine in an herbalomic base

#188 TMI LIQUID—This formula nourishes and supports the thyroid metabolic processes via multi-source iodine in an herbalomic base

#192 CALMD LIQUID—BONE SUPP + VITD—Supports healthy aging bones utilizing a unique blend of calcium, magnesium, strontium, boron and zinc; plus vitamin K2 and collagen for healthy bones.

#195 ZNC-ZINC CHELATE—This formula is a valuable, natural source of zinc which is the key to support healthy digestive enzymes, reproductive organ development and the proper production of hormones

#197 OMGA LQ—OMEGA 3, 6, 9 LIQUID—This is an ultra pure essential fatty acid (Omega 3, 6 & 9) formula that supports healthy heart, brain and joint function.

#199 VITD3 LQ—VITD3 + K2 LIQUID COMPLEX—Clinically effective supplement for establishing activated vitamin D receptors associated with optimal health

BIO EXTRACT—containing the active ingredient of a substance in concentrated form

#200 AO-ALOE VERA—A 4-times concentration of Aloe Vera extracted from the inner gel (inside the leaves). For internal and topical applications.

#210 CA-CATS-A-TONIC—This herbal extract combines the Cat's Claw herb. Supports healthy immune function.

#225 EE-ESSENCE OIL—An essential oil formula most often used topically as an analgesic for muscles and joints. Supports muscle comfort, and healthy skin color.

#241 EV-ELIXER VITA—An herbal extract that boosts energy, nutritionally assists the immune system and cleansing.

#243 IA-IMPERIAL ATAKER—The liquid form of the famous ATAK (Immune Rejuvenator) formula that addresses immunological support

#245 RV-RENOVATOR—Effectively moisturizes and brings relief to dry, chapped and/or sunburned skin.

#250 TR-TAI RA CHI 2oz—Immune support plus an ultra-high energy cellular support, derived from polarity-corrected Brazilian Pau D'Arco. Helpful when dealing with issues associated with temporary immune disturbance.

#254 TR-TAI RA CHI 1oz—Immune support plus an ultra-high energy cellular support, derived from polarity-corrected Brazilian Pau D'Arco. Helpful when dealing with issues associated with temporary immune disturbance.

#260 WO-CHINA HEALING OIL—Essential oil combination "medicine chest" in a bottle.

#270 SC-CLEANSER—Proanthocyanidin-rich (antioxidant) extract formula comes from fermented grapefruit rind and is a topical application for temporary skin issues.

#298 COLD-ZINCA STOP—Large amounts of zinc have been shown to block cold viruses from adhering to the nasal lining and/or replicating themselves

BIOME—naturally occurring community of flora in the body

#350 ECO-VIRMOE—Kills Ecoli—designed to support the proliferation of beneficial bacteria throughout the gastrointestinal tract. Prebioitic phage

#360 MUSCLE REJUVENATION—microbiota friendly hot and cool formula to help manage aches, pains and other muscle and joint stress

#375 PSEUDO-VIROME—Kills pseudomonus aeruginosa. Prebiotic phage.

#379 SKIN COLONIZER—recolonizes the skin with good bacteria. Great for rashes, eczema, psoriasis, and other skin coniditions.

#380 SAL-VIROME—Kills salmonella—help maintain a normal and healthy gastrointestinal system. prebioitic phage. Great for situations of food poisoning.

BIO CHALLENGE—a call to challenge the body

#400 APHA-PH CONTROL—supports a healthful pH value and healthful "ebb and flow" of pH cycles

#402 ARTA-JOINT—Provides natural botanical and biochemical support for healthy joints, comfort, and daily physical stress

#403 ATAK-IMMUNE REJUVENATOR—immunological support from the unique stand point of transporting essential botanical factors with rapid assimilation to support immunological response.

#404 BIND-TOXIN ELIMINATION—provides toxin and heavy metal binding matrices such as activated carbon and purified humates to support natural toxin elimination.

#405 BLDB—By combining bovine tissue factors from the liver, kidney and spleen with purified hemablobin and herbalomic factors the formula creates the perfect base for nutrients consumed in the production of healthy blood chemistry.

#406 CALM-STRESS RELIEF—nutrients that play a role in the synthesis of neurotransmitters, such as serotonin and dopamine with L-Dopa and SAMe.

#408 CLNZ-CHELATOR—A traditional gentle chelation and cleansing formula

#425 DIJS-ACIDEZE—DIJS Promotes stomach and esophageal comfort via Potassium Bitartrate.

#427 DREM-SLEEP AID—Formulated to promote a restful, relaxed state and relieve occasional sleeplessness by beneficially modulating the metabolism of melatonin and promoting relaxation.

#428 DSIR-INTERGEN—Formulated to support the Stomach-Duodenal-Thyroid triad which is foundational to health in Traditional Chinese Medicine.

#433 GCEL-INTRACELLULAR GLUTATHIONE—boost the body's production of glutathione peroxidase, a primary antioxidant throughout the entire body. Protects the body against oxidative stress and detoxifying harmful compounds.

#435 GOLD-IMMUNE PLUS—very powerful immune support that operates through a complex process of providing cellular stain markers that interact with bacterial communications as well as supporting the immune response.

#450 KDIR-FLUIDREN—Helps with water retentiveness, normal kidney fuction, and normal kidney mideral sediment processes

#460 KYRO-MUSCLE, TISSUE, LIGAMENT—Support for ligaments, muscles and tissues. Helpful in promoting comfort post exercise.

#467 LGUT-LEAKY GUT MASTERY—Reparis intestinal and stomach tissues. Support the intestinal mucosa by up-regulating the tight junction protein claudin and down-regulating the protein zonulin.

#481 OXAA-ORGANIZER CELL—This formula was designed as a support for deep tissue detoxificiation processes such as those involving liver, bones, breasts and prostate.

#482 OXCC-CLEANSER CELL—This herbal formula supports ATP energy processes for cellular cleansing processes. It supports already healthy cell function and development.

#483 OXOX-ACTIVATOR CELL—Cleansing of deep tissue and lymphatic drainage, and broad based blood cleansing herbal protocols.

#486 SENG-LYMPHOGIN—This herbal, "American Ginseng" formula helps support the lymphatic system and the flow of lymphatic fluids throughout the body

#488 VIVI-VIROX—Viral Killer. Clinical Doses of Lomatium dissecutim and Pau D' Arco

#491 VRM1-LARGE—Kills large parasitic organisms

#492 VRM2-SMALL—Kills small parasitic organisms

#493 VRM3-MICRO—Kills microscopic parasitic organisms

#494 VRM4-CELL—Kills cellular parasitic organisms

KIDZ PLAY—products made specifically for children and teens

#508 BONEZ PLAY-BONE BUILDER + VIT D3—Children and teen bone health

#510 BRAINY PLAY—OMEGA 3, 6 & 9—support healthy heart, brain, and nervous system development in children.

#520 FUN PLAY—MULTI VITAMIN MINERAL—Nutritionally balanced formula of vitamins, antioxidants, minerals and botanicals to support children's everyday health and wellness.

#530 TUFF PLAY—ESSENTIAL IMMUNE BOOST—supports children's healthy immune function.

BIO BASIC—essential foundation and starting point for the body; fundamentals

#610 ACCELL THERAPEUTIC—smoothy powder provides potent nutritional support as the foundation for every natural health program, especially when used in detoxification programs.

#613 COLLAGEN ECM—Supports skin, tendons, joints, bones, organs, cartilage, fibers, and hair (no taste powder and dissolves well)

#620 METABO SHAKE BERRY/GREENS—highly potent metabolic formula which provides a pure macro and micro nutrient profile. Includes greens like kale, spinach, and broccoli. Great for weight management and metabolic support.

#625 METABO SHAKE CHOCOLATE—highly potent metabolic formula which provides a pure macro and micro nutrient profile. Great for weight management and metabolic support.

#630 METABO SHAKE VANILLA—highly potent metabolic formula which provides a pure macro and micro nutrient profile. Great for weight management and metabolic support.

#660 MELA—OPTIMAL TERRAIN ENZYMES—protease enzymes in an herbalomic base focused on protein breakdown for optimal absorption.

#650 ENZEE-HI POTENCY ENZYMES—A potent herb-based formula containing highly effective enzymes that focus on carbohydrate breakdown.

#637 ZGLUTN-GLUTEN CONTROL ENZYMES—This formula is a combination of concentrated enzymes and herbs designed to support the digestion of gluten and casein.

CHINESE 5 ELEMENTS—the five elements of Qi.

#720 GENERAL SEDATE—Relieve Depression and Invigorate Vitality—This formula is the 'Great Energy Balancer'; it supports feelings of inner peace, confidence, patience, and calm

#725 GENERAL TONIFY—Generate the Pulse—This formula tonifies, strengthens and nourishes the lungs, spleen, kidneys, and liver. It tonifies Qi and yang.

#730 ENERGY SEDATE—Clear Heat—This formula promotes healthy function of the throat, skin, lymph, and eyes. It clears and balances heat and drains fire thereby cooling layers, and nourishes yin.

#735 ENERGY TONIFY—Tonify Yin—designed to tone the body's structure including the bones, nerves, skin, lymph, and eyes. This is a cooling, rest-promoting, and nourishing formula

#740 EARTH SEDATE—Clear Congestion—supports balance of the digestive system. The earth element is often associated with nutrition—the digestion and assimilation of what the earth brings forth and the incorporation of it into the bod

#745 EARTH TONIFY—Warm the Center—important in helping people care for themselves as well as others both physically and emotionally. Clinicians often use this formula to accompany healthy weight programs.

#750 FIRE SEDATE—Pacify the Spirit—this formula is for people who've lost their boundaries, who are over-exuberant, over stimulated, and overly excited or overly excitable

#755 FIRE TONIFY—Support the Heart—heart symptoms, congestive concerns, overly serious, melancholy, lonely, shy, blood pressure high or low, anemic,

#760 METAL SEDATE—Ventilate the Lungs—designed as a support for the respiratory system. It supports peaceful breathing, lung and respiratory functions for overallhealth.

#765 METAL TONIFY—Support the Weak and Thin—designed to support lung, throat, spleen and large intestine health.

#770 WATER SEDATE—Remove Dampness—this formula supports the kidneys, spleen and digestion

#775 WATER TONIFY—Strengthen Bones—This formula supports the health of bones, kidneys, spleen, digestive system, and connective tissues.

#780 WOOD SEDATE—Mediate Harmony—This formula supports the health of the liver, blood, spleen and digestion.

#785 WOOD TONIFY—Tonify Blood—this product may help nourish liver-blood; enrich kidney's yin and subdue yang

BIO CELL—supports the cellular level of the body

#810 ENRG-QUANTUM CELLULAR ATP ENERGY—Supplies key nutrients for the mitochondrial production of ATP

#811 ENRG LQ-QUANTUM CELLULAR ATP ENERGY LQ—Supplies key nutrients for the mitochondrial production of ATP

#820 EPIC-METABOLIC ANTIOXIDANT—Micro antioxidant to reduce inflammation of the cells. Supports the NO/ONOO cycle.

#821 EPIC LQ-METABOLIC ANTIOXIDANT LQ—Micro antioxidant to reduce inflammation of the cells. Supports the NO/ONOO cycle.

#840 EVENTA-CELLULAR ENZYME CORRECTOR—Supports optimal cellular function of the many Nitric Oxide Synthase (NOS) pathways. Male hormone support. Support muscle integrity, organ and gland health, and increased energy.

#841 EVENTA LQ-CELL ENZYME CORRECTOR LQ—Supports optimal cellular function of the many Nitric Oxide Synthase (NOS) pathways. Male hormone support. Support muscle integrity, organ and gland health, and increased energy.

#843 FEMICRINE-FEMALE ENDOCRINE SUPPORT—Positively influences cellular status, healthy estrogen activity, feminine microbiome and breast health.

#850 MORS-METHYLATION DONOR—Behavior Support (Positive Mood), Energy, Stress Management. Providing the L-5-methyltetrahydrofolate form of folate.

#851 MORS LQ-METHYLATION DONOR LQ—Behavior Support (Positive Mood), Energy, Stress Management. Providing the L-5-methyltetrahydrofolate form of folate.

#854 NEUROSYN-NEURO COGNITIVE MEMORY SUPPORT—formulated to support healthy brain aging, cognition, and memory by beneficially modulating the metabolism of the neurotransmitter acetylcholine and providing neuroprotection.

#865 RPM—Pro-Resolvin, Protectin, Maresin—formulated to provide the body nutritional EPA/DHA, plus synergistic White Willow Extract to support the resolving phase of the natural inflammation activities.

#870 SPECTRA 1-WHOLE FOOD MULTI VIT—100% certified organic, plant-based, full-spectrum (synergists included) Multi Vitamin/Mineralsupplement.

#871 SPECTRA 1 LIQUID—100% certified organic, plant-based, full-spectrum (synergists included) Multi Vitamin/Mineralsupplement.

#872 SPECTRA 2 OIL—comprehensive, plant-sourced, nutritional oilsupplement due to the select blend and inclusion of rare Omega fatty acids that present the body with a wide array offatty acids for cellular, molecular use.

#875 SYNULIN-GLYCEMIC BALANCE—assists insulin in the biochemical regulation of fat, carbohydrate, and protein metabolism

#880 VISTA 1-MEMBRANE REGENERATION—supports cell membrane integrity via essential phospholipids, antioxidants, amino acids, and botanicals.

#881 VISTA 1 LQ-MEMBRANE REGENERATION—supports cell membrane integrity via essential phospholipids, antioxidants, amino acids, and botanicals.

#882 VISTA 2-MEMBRANE REGENERATION OIL—supports cell membrane integrity via essential phospholipids, antioxidants, amino acids, and botanicals.

#883 VISTA 2-MEMBRANE REGENERATION GELCAPS—supports cell membrane integrity via essential phospholipids, antioxidants, amino acids, and botanicals.

BIO TINCTURE—18.18% less potency than the original formulation

#1003 T3-BACTREX TINCTURE—Kills bacteria and helps the production of white blood cells

#1004 T4-FUNGDX TINCTURE—Kills fungus and slows fungal growth

#1005 T5-STABILIZER TINCTURE—Supports proper cellular reproduction and stabalizes functions in the body

#1102 TACX-VITAMIN DTX TINCTURE—High potency, broad-spectrum detoxifier; an excellent drainage formula for use in any cleansing, eliminationprogram, and/or detoxification program, especially for organ detoxification

#1435 TGOLD-IMMUNE PLUS TINCTURE—very powerful immune support that operates through a complex process of providing cellular stain markers that interact with bacterial communications as well as supporting the immune response.

#1488 TVIVI-VIROX TINCTURE—Viral Killer. Clinical Doses of Lomatium dissecutim and Pau D' Arco

CX EXTRACTS—concentrated liquid options

#2001 CX1—ACTIVATOR—Provides nutrients that support hypothalamic functions

#2002 CX2—BUILDER—Supports tissues' inherent rebuilding function

#2003 CX3—BACTREX—Kills bacteria and helps the production of white blood cells

#2004 CX4—FUNGDX—Kills fungus and slows fungal growth

#2005 CX5—STABALIZER—Supports proper cellular reproduction and stabalizes functions in the body

#2006 CX6—RESTORE—Nutrients support cellular integrity and restores fuctions in the body

#2012 CXB—BRAIN—Nourishes the neuronal cellular matrix; supports the brain's normal processes of concentration

#2022 CXF+—FEMALE PLUS—Provides nutritional support for healthy female biochemistry, hormonal balance and ovarian/uterine health.

#2024 CXFPMS—FEMALE HEALTH—Support to help normalize the menstrual cycle associated with excessive bleeding, hot flashes, mood swings and accompanying dysmenorrhea cramps.

#2031 CXGA—ADRENAL—Builds and balances the adrenal glands

#2032 CXGB—PITUITARY/PINEAL—Provides nutritional support for all the important brain glands—pituitary, pineal, and thalamus

#2039 CXGF—THYROID—Builds and balances the thyroid gland

#2041 CXGT—THYMUS—Provides the perfect nutrition for the thymus gland, the immune system's master regulator

#2044 CXH—HEART—Provides nutrients for optimal heart health to strengthen the heart muscle

#2050 CXI—EYES—Supports the brain's optic center (back lobes); supplies nutrients necessary for clear vision

#2056 CXK—KIDNEY—Kidney support formula for integrity of the kidney tissue. K Kidney is also a great addition to a general bladder health protocol.

#2060 CXL—LIVER—Liver building formula that supports building & maintenance of the liver's intercellular tissues

#2061 CXLB—LIVER/GALL BLADDER—Designed for general liver/gallbladder support and cleansing. Helps the body maintain proper portal duct function.

#2062 CXLS—LIVER S—Supports the liver's function and provides nutrient cofactors consumed in the liver's innate detoxification processes

#2070 CXM+—MALE ENDOCRINE—Supports the male glandular and endocrine systems

#2072 CXMPC—PROSTATA CORRECTOR—Prostate support formula that provides nutritional factors that support a healthy prostate gland and healthy circulation

#2074 CXN—NERVE—General nerve support for the whole nervous system with specific herbalomic nutriments for nerve support for the bundle branch nerves that serve the heart

#2075 CXN3—RELAXA—Designed for individuals who have feelings of anxiety and disorientation and have difficulty resting due to occasional stress; N3 provides nutrients that support the calming neurtransmitter response of GABA

#2077 CXNC—CALM—nutrients that play a role in the synthesis of neurotransmitters, such as serotonin and dopamine with L-Dopa and SAMe.

#2078 CXP—PANCREAS—Supports normal pancreatic functions including production of insulin & glucagons and tissue integrity

#2080 CXR—LUNG—Complete Nutritional Lung support. This formula was designed to support a healthy respiratory system and maintain normal mucus levels, as well as to support the oxygen-carrying capacity of the lungs

#2082 CXS—SPLEEN—Nutritional support for the spleen. Supports spleen health which can influence the lymphatic and blood systems as well as the immune system

#2102 CXACX—VITAMIN DTX—High potency, broad-spectrum detoxifier; an excellent drainage formula for use in any cleansing, elimination program, and/or detoxification program, especially for organ detoxification

#2400 CXAPHA—PH CONTROL—supports a healthful pH value and healthful "ebb and flow" of pH cycles

#2408 CXCLNZ—CHELATOR—A traditional gentle chelation and cleansing formula

#2435 CXGOLD—IMMUNE PLUS—very powerful immune support that operates through a complex process of providing cellular stain markers that interact with bacterial communications as well as supporting the immune response.

#2481 CXOXAA—ORGANIZER CELL—This formula was designed as a support for deep tissue detoxificiation processes such as those involving liver, bones, breasts and prostate.

#2482 CXOXCC—CLEANSER CELL—This herbal formula supports ATP energy processes for cellular cleansing processes. It supports already healthy cell function and development.

#2482 CXOXOX—ACTIVATOR CELL—Cleansing of deep tissue and lymphatic drainage, and broad based blood cleansing herbal protocols.

#2486   CXSENG—LYMPHOGIN—This herbal, "American Ginseng" formula helps support the lymphatic system and the flow of lymphatic fluids throughout the body

#2488 CXVIVI—VIROX—Viral Killer. Clinical Doses of Lomatium dissecutim and Pau D' Arco

#2491 CXVRM1—LARGE—Kills large parasitic organisms

#2492 CXVRM2—SMALL—Kills small parasitic organisms

#2493 CXVRM3—MICRO—Kills microscopic parasitic organisms

#2494 CXVRM4—CELL—Kills cellular parasitic organisms

PROGRAM PACKAGES

#916 IDS PACKAGE—This package provides cutting edge glutathione support for true cellular detoxification

#920 CORE CELLULAR PACKAGE—This program addresses the clinical health at the cellular level. It's based in the premise of the 5-R's of clinical support, stating that if you support the cell, the body can maintain optimal health

#925 DETOX PACKAGE—This 3-phase, 60-day package offers safe, effective and complete liver support, comprehensive drainage, neuroendocrine system and cellular function support.

#930 GI PURGE PACKAGE—This package supports the cleansing processes of the GI tract.

#934 GI WELLNESS PACKAGE—This package supports G.I. health, functions, promotes healthy microbiome terrain, supports tight junctions and recolonizes the G.I. system with healthy bacteria

#940 CELL DETOX BODY PHASE—Detoxes the cells in the body of chemicals, heavy metals, and other toxins

#941 CELL DETOX BRAIN PHASE—Detoxes the brain cells of chemicals, heavy metals, and other toxins

#942 CELLULAR VITALITY PHASE—Replenishes the cells with nutrients

#943 CELL DETOX PREP PHASE—Prepares the body for cellular detoxification

#950 THYROID PACKAGE—This program supports the thyroids cellular metabolism, nourishes the thyroid and adrenal tissues. Provides tissue specific anti-oxidant nutrients.

#3090 MUSCLE & JOINT REJUVENATION—Our "Inside-Out Outside-In" nutritional topical and oral therapy is designed to provide broad support for healthy joints and muscle soft tissue by providing high quality nutrition.

As I mentioned before, I also wanted to share with you about an area on your feet, for I have found this area to be quite tender and can be extremely painful on those who are suffering acutely from illnesses of any kind which includes headaches, migraines, injuries, energy blocks, sleep issues and the list goes on. This is the one and only area in the body that just seems to tackle any and all issues and especially those of you who have trouble sleeping and headaches.

CAUTION!!! IF YOU ARE PREGNANT DO NOT WORK (PALPATE) THIS SPOT
THIS IS AN EXTREMLY POWERFUL AREA

Unless you are working directly with an acupuncturist

For there are certain points on the body that are known to Induce labor!!

**Palpating: is like tapping with a finger, except you do not break contact with the skin. I have found if I do break contact with the skin, then I'm not ever able to release the tenderness from the acupressure point. I always use my middle fingertip (which is considered *the fire finger* in Chinese Medicine)

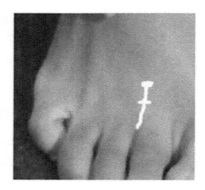

This area lays just off the edge of the stomach meridian *(you can look up Chinese meridians on line to view where they flow through the body)* so when you are a trying to find the point to relieve the tenderness, for those of you who are not familiar with body work at all these instructions are for you and you will want to be very careful as to not over stimulate the area! *(this is why I urge people to take a class or have someone who understands how to do acupressure treatments to show you how to palpate you can also search utube)* you will start at the base between the second and third toes, using your thumb or middle finger start by walking it gently towards the ankle *(remember this area*

can be extremely painful so I caution you to go very gentle when pressing if it's not so sensitive you may press a bit harder till the person feels the tenderness) when the person you are helping starts to feel the tenderness, then go one more finger width towards the ankle or until you are on the most painful spot within the area as I have marked in the photo. Then that's when you want to palpate the tender spot for no more than a minute this is very important so as not to over stimulate causing more issues for the person you are helping. You may do this treatment two to three times a day till the point starts to feel better and all the pain has been released. When I have done this treatment for clients who are very ill, it has taken me up to a week at times for the point to finally release completely, then after it releases I continue to check every day to see if there is any tenderness and if so then I will palpate it up to a minute until the tenderness is gone. After you have released all the pain clear to the bone, then you may want to check it every day and then every other day or two and so on, as you would a wound to make sure there is no infection setting in. You want this area to be kept pain free which in turn may help immensely a speedier recovery of the friend or loved one you are helping.

I must also share with you that when I recently started using the WO oil on these acupressure points, surprisingly enough the pain started to diminish! So I've started applying the WO oil to the top of my foot, a drop on the bottom of both feet, the inside of my knees, and above the ankle on the inside of the leg as well as.

Tip: *To use for an all over Body Lotion I add a few drops to a small bottle of olive oil, coconut oil or even avocado oil and then be sure to shake well before each use. This is very important to do as to not to cause a painful skin rash from the essential oils.*

There are so many bodywork tips I'd love to share with you! So that's why Dr. Troy Crane and I are putting a class together for those of you that would like to learn some hands-on, self-help techniques you can use to help you and your family with.

————Ask us about coming to your area————
You will find the contact information for classes at the end of this book.

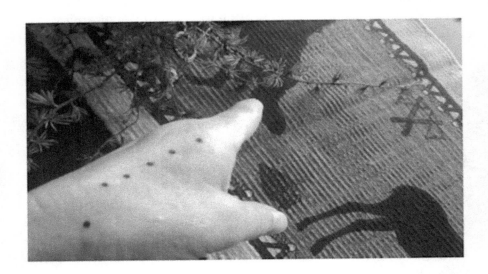

Illustration 1: Headache points: Illustration 1: The black dots on the hand are areas I palpate for headaches, migraines and when someone just doesn't feel well. These points are on the bone, not in the muscles. I search for the most tender points and then palpate them. I find that just rubbing them will not help dissipate the pain. I will generally check this area everyday for tenderness.

*How to massage your ileocecal valve: Go to the right of your navel approximately three finger widths and then down towards the hip approximately two inches, basically half way between your navel and top of your hip. When you press into your abdomen a bit you will feel a tightness and most likely tenderness. The more issues you have with digestion, the more tender or right down painful it is.

Now that you have found your ileocecal valve, while pressing into your abdomen make a clock-wise motion two or three times then release instantly *(as quickly as you can)* you may do this a couple of times. If it is easier you may also just palpate the most tender spot till you feel it relax a bit, this may take a minute. Then you can press in and rotate that tender spot a couple of times clock-wise then let go of it by releasing it quickly.

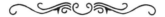

By palpating an inch from all corners and sides of the navel may help help keep valves more relaxed allowing the organs and lymphatics to drain more efficiently. I generally do this in the morning before getting out of bed and then at night after going to bed while lying on my back. In a week's time you should start noticing that your abdomen isn't as tight as it was before starting this treatment. Remember it is very important to not over due the treatments!! You can detox yourself to much to fast…THEN YOU CAN GET YOURSELF IN MORE TROUBLE. Like the guy I worked on a few times with backed up lymphatics in his left leg due to a tumor growing in his left hip. The last time I saw him he told me he had decided to purchase a lymphatic pump for his ankle to keep his lymph's moving. He then proceeded to lift his shirt up to show me his liver which had swollen clear out from under his ribs it was very tight looking resembling much like a watermelon! He said "that happened after he put the lymphatic pump around his ankle and then accidentally fell asleep for TWO HOURS!"

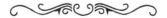

Tip *for massaging: when massaging your abdomen always go in a clock-wise direction so as not to back the colon up by starting on your right side moving to the left. The reason I thought I would mentioned this, is that I've actually had clients who came to see about their digestion issues they would mention to me and show me how they would try to help their digestion by massaging their abdomen and yes, you guessed it they were going backwards on their colon most likely causing constipation among other issues and not feeling well in-general.*

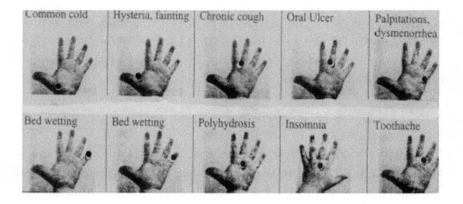

** I inserted this hand chart to give you some extra points to release and to apply WO oil as well, which may help in these instances listed in this chart. As I mentioned before, when working acupressure points, palpate points on both hands or feet the same amount of time. Plus if you are doing acupressure for someone else then work the same point on both sides of the body at the same time.

Bodywork is a very powerful tool to help the body on it's healing journey, although just like any other tool whether it be a steak knife or a garden tool, they all have to be treated and used with the proper respect.

For further information about classes for my Nerve Tissue Release Technique among other helpful treatments such as my reinvented easy reflexology treatment, visit my website you may contact me by email, phone call or text, if no answer please leave a message, I will be happy to return your call as soon as I can.

CONCLUSION

I pray, my story will help inspire you *that* there is help out there.

May peace be in your heart, and the Good Lord be with you and Bless you always with Love, Good Health, and Abundance! And thank you once again for sharing your time with me!

Most truly,
Kathy Gaa, ND, LMT, CBCP

To order products and for more information about treatments (modalities) and products, I welcome you to visit my website at www. mountainrosewellnesscenter.com

I am petitioning all Body-Workers who have these skills, and who are "passionately dedicated" in helping and learning "my format" to help battle against Lyme & West Nile, you may send your business contact information to me. I will add you to a business directory on my website for the people who are looking for a Therapist in their area that uses the modalities listed above.
Lets Work as a Team to Help Fight the battle of pain and suffering from Lyme and West Nile.

***Disclaimer: *No representation contained in these materials is intended as medical advice and should not be used for diagnosis or medical treatments.*

My Contact Information:

Email: kathygaa@gmail.com or you may go to my website to email me.
kathy@mountainrosewellnesscenter.com

Phone: 208.223.9875
Office Hours: 11:00 am to 4:00 pm MST (Mountain Standard Time)

ABOUT THE AUTHOR

The year is 2020, I am writing this book to share with you my experiences and the battles I have had and how I am now finally winning the battle with Lyme and West-nile, and finally able to see more clearly just how God has used these diseases and the paths he directed me on to meet the gifted, Instructors, Doctors, as well as those naturally gifted healers, who also came into my life that helped in so many ways, which in turn helped me to inspire, and offer help others on their healing path as well.

There are various challenges and troubles each and every one of us has to encounter in life. You will sometimes discover that people show concern toward assisting you. As lovely as this may possibly sound, you are the only one that can take that first step to helping yourself.

That is if you actually care enough to begin the journey to help yourself.

This is my story and I pray it will be an inspiration to live a healthier life. *Thank you for this time to share in your life!*

CPSIA information can be obtained
at www.ICGtesting.com
Printed in the USA
BVHW081243221221
624595BV00006B/801